GOODBYE
LUPUS

How a Medical Doctor Healed Herself
Naturally With Supermarket Foods

BROOKE GOLDNER, M.D.

Brooke Goldner, M.D
Published by Express Results, LLC Austin, TX

First Edition 2015

Important Legal Notice And Disclaimer:
This publication is intended to provide educational information with regard to the
subject matter covered.
The reader of this book assumes all responsibility for the use of these materials and
information Brooke Goldner, M.D. and Express Results, LLC assume no responsibility or
liability whatsoever on behalf of any purchaser or reader of these materials.
The methodology, training, products, mentoring, or other teaching does not guarantee
success and the results may vary.
The information in this book should not substitute for medical care by a licensed
practitioner.
Please notify your doctor about any nutritional or alternative therapy you intend to use.

Table of Contents

Author's Note

In this book, I hope to be able to give you information on my battle with Lupus and how anyone afflicted by the disease can go on! Life doesn't have to stop because of Lupus.

I want you to know my story because this was never supposed to happen. Everything I was told as a sick child, and my 16 years of experience in the medical field said this wasn't supposed to happen, but it did.

Modern research has shown that most diseases that are killing Americans each and every day are treatable and sometimes even reversible through proper diet. Modern medical schools have not caught up with this idea and haven't yet begun to endorse it.

As a doctor, I have patients reaching out to me on a daily basis asking how to regain their health and get off the medications they have been taking.

You, too, can be healthier and live better than you ever realized was possible!

It is my hope that I will be able to help you do this.

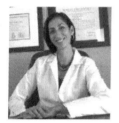

My Early Life and Childhood

When I was a child, I was very privileged as we had our own personal chef. He was famous and enjoyed by many children and adults alike. You've probably heard of him; his name is Chef Boyardee.

Mom loved me so much that she made sure I had a warm thermos full of my favorite canned pasta dishes for lunch at school every day.

My grandmother would watch me after school, and she was always willing to serve up some boxed macaroni and cheese. I thought homemade mac' and cheese was disgusting; I needed the stuff that came in the blue box with the powdered cheese! I suppose some of us children are funny that way.

While I had also always enjoyed munching on a raw tomatoes, cucumbers, apples, and bananas; processed, canned, and boxed foods were a large part of my daily diet during my childhood.

In my teen years, I hit the jackpot in ways that only a teenager can truly appreciate. My dad had decided to buy a pizza franchise. He sold his pizza to the school lunch program as a fresher and healthier alternative to the frozen pizza squares they had been selling us. This was a huge bonus for me as it meant pizza all day long!

I wasn't much of a water drinker as a kid. Back then, I believed that water was something that you drank if you didn't have the money for soda or other drinks. They hadn't yet come out with bottled water and I remember poking fun at the ridiculous idea of paying for water when bottled water started being sold in stores.

At home, I drank the diet soda my mother had stocked the fridge with. I drank "real soda" the sugary stuff when we went to a restaurant.

Despite my processed eating habits, I was fortunate to be naturally skinny no matter what I ate. While I was always a very thin child, I was completely unathletic. I preferred reading, writing poetry and songs, and anything cerebral to anything physical. Since I was thin and looked fairly healthy, I was encouraged to eat whatever I wanted. No one had any reason to believe otherwise.

I know I wasn't the only student who would do anything they could to get out of taking gym class. Sports seemed pointless to me and also fairly dangerous whenever a ball was being thrown in my direction. I swear there is a magnetic current that runs from airborne balls straight to my head! Even by the time I graduated from high school, I couldn't complete the mile run that we had to attempt once a year in gym class without walking and gasping for air. Despite my poor results on the yearly Presidential Fitness Challenges, I could get around to my classes just fine and lift up my backpack without too much effort, so I guess I appeared fit enough.

Looking back now, I can easily see how obvious it was that my body was being set-up for illness. Between the poor foods and lack of physical activity, it was unhealthy and potentially dangerous. However, back then if you were thin and energetic, which I was, you were considered healthy.

My family truly did think they were showing me love by giving me the foods I enjoyed. I know that they only wanted what was good for me and never had any malicious intent toward me. Despite this line of thought, a lot of harm can come from well-intentioned people. Think of it as that cliché of "the road to hell is paved with good intentions." Along this line of thinking, I have talked to some parents who thought it was "mean" to give their children plain water instead of juice or soda because it doesn't taste good. How many of you still consider fast food and ice cream a treat rather than a toxin?

Ignorance is not bliss and the lack of knowledge can be dangerous. I encourage you to read on with an open mind. The long-term benefits will be far greater than the short-term displeasure of having to make some changes.

My Illness

It was a complete shock to my family and myself when I was diagnosed with Lupus when I was just 16 years old. It can be truly earth shattering when you are diagnosed with a disease. My world was broken when I went from a world where I could do anything to a world where I couldn't.

Before my diagnosis, I was a great student, active in yearbook, and even played on the volleyball team. Okay, so that isn't entirely true, as I sat on the bench for the volleyball team. I did have a uniform, though! I had an active social life and enjoyed staying up late at sleepovers and spending my summers with friends at the shore.

The symptoms started gradually, with arthritis being the first symptom. When the arthritis started, I convinced myself I must have been overdoing it at volleyball and general physical activity. Considering my rather sedentary life that seems a bit silly to me now, but my mind tried to find simple explanations for physical discomforts. Still, the arthritis progressed. There would be days when I would be trying to write in class and it was so hard to hold the pen because the joints in my fingers were so painful and stiff. Other days I would be limping up the steps on achy knees trying to get to my class on time. My knees would be so weak and painful that I would have to take breaks in the middle of the stairwell or hold on to something to make it up the two flights of stairs.

I told my parents about the pains and they said, "That's strange, let's make an appointment to the doctor." Despite the call, I would have to wait to have my appointment and all sorts of other things began to happen in the meantime.

I was at the Jersey shore for a weekend in the summer. My friends and I had gone to the beach to play volleyball. While I was not good on the court, if I were in the sand with people who did not know how to play volleyball, I had some serious moves! I remember diving in the sand and spiking the ball. I was having a great day.

After a long day and night, we were walking along the boardwalk, talking, gossiping, and laughing. We all got up probably around 2:00pm the following afternoon, and were going to the diner for a very late breakfast.

I remember that day so clearly because I woke up with the most excruciating pain in my right shoulder. This was the worst pain I had ever experienced. I honestly didn't even know it was humanly possible to feel pain on that level.

I sat at the diner with my friends who were giggling and chatting and here I was having trouble lifting my arm to get pancakes into my mouth. I wanted to cry but didn't, especially not in front of my friends.

I didn't know what was going on or what was wrong with me. I blamed the pain on the moves I had done the previous day. I must have been spiking that ball a bit too hard. Still, this pain went beyond muscle soreness, and I decided I was going to tell my mom when I got home because I didn't know if I had broken anything. Maybe I'd go to the doctor for an X-ray.

The next day, when I woke up, the pain in my right shoulder wasn't there. I thought to myself, *That's strange. A pain that severe should take days...maybe weeks to heal.* But even stranger, now the exact same excruciating pain was in my left shoulder. How could that happen?

If anyone has ever had migrating joint pain, they know it can be a very confusing thing. I had begun to wonder and question my own memory. I remember thinking to myself, "Okay, wait, I know it was in my right shoulder... the fork for the pancakes was in my right hand; the syrup was in my left hand, fork in the right hand... It was the right shoulder. Right shoulder! Now it's the left one and the same thing. Was it really the right shoulder?" I just couldn't figure it out. It just didn't make sense.

Since it was very confusing to me, I didn't tell anyone. It didn't make sense to me so how could it make sense to anyone else? What was I going to tell Mom? "Hi Mom, I, like, really threw out my right shoulder but it's better now. But the pain moved to my left shoulder." So I left the subject alone and didn't discuss it. For some reason that made sense to my teenage mind.

I even broke out into a weird rash on my face. It was a bright red rash on both of my cheeks and over the bridge of my nose. I soon learned it was called a butterfly rash. Being 16, I reasoned that complexion issues were something every teenager went through, and I just used makeup to cover it up.

The straw that broke the camel's back was the migraines. I started getting so many migraines, and they would be so bad that I would be bent over a bucket or the toilet and vomiting up the contents of my stomach for two days straight before they started to subside.

Many years later, I was telling my mom that I was giving the keynote speech for an event by Lupus LA. When we started talking about the early days of my illness, she started crying. She began to tell me stories that I didn't even remember.

She told me that one day we were out for dinner with my friends and family when I was struck with a migraine. I became so sick she had to take me home and leave everyone else there. She even had to keep pulling the car over so I could lean out the car door and vomit.

I have no memory of the incident, but she remembered it clearly. It struck me then and it even strikes me now that I think our families suffer with us when we are sick, and how they sometimes suffer much more than we do. There were times I would see them crying and I'd think, *but I'm doing okay.* I will never forget the sight of my grandmother on her knees wailing up at the ceiling asking God to take her instead of me.

One day, I got home from a day at the pool with my friend, and I had an awful migraine. After vomiting, I sat down wearily beside my father at the kitchen table, and he saw the bright rash on my face. He told me that he thought the skin was the window to your health and that something must be seriously wrong. I remember rolling my eyes at his "Dad Science." We always joked around that my dad had his own Dad Science that came from his head and wasn't necessarily scientific at all. It turns out that Dad had it right this time. It's funny because now I teach my clients the same thing – the skin *is* the window to your health!

Extremely concerned, my parents called my doctor and told her the whole list of what was going on. They were immediately told, "Meet me in the ER."

Isn't it funny and incredible how something can be so horribly wrong, and our brains will try to make it seem like normal problems? There are times our brains look for simple answers and this was one of them. Being young, and not understanding what was wrong with my body, I was doing my best to rationalize what could be causing this. How bad could it be? My poor family, however, were probably near hysterics in not knowing what was wrong with me.

We met my doctor in the ER and she immediately ordered blood work. They took seven tubes of blood from me! I was going to run out of blood samples if this continued! I couldn't recall ever having blood work before and I was freaked out when I saw that needle! It took two nurses to hold me down and a third to do the blood draw!

All of this just to get some blood work. I actually remember by the end of the second week of my diagnosis, I would go in for blood tests and sit for the needle without even flinching. It had become nothing to me. It had already become routine. That's kind of sad within itself, isn't it?

The diagnosis was also far worse than I ever imagined it could be. Not only did I have arthritis, rashes, and migraines, my blood tests indicated kidney disease and I would have to undergo an urgent kidney biopsy.

The diagnosis was terrifying – I had the most aggressive form of Lupus nephritis! They called it severe Systemic Lupus Erythematosus. To make matters worse, my kidneys would most likely fail completely in six months if they didn't intervene in a powerful way! It's better known as type IV Nephritis. Kidney failure. Not good. Not good at all.

My poor family. They had gone from having this healthy wonderful child to "our child could die" overnight. What a horrible and terrible realization to have dumped on you without even so much as a warning. While my mother stayed strong to my face, I can still remember hearing her cry behind her bedroom door at night. I will never forget seeing my grandmother on her knees begging God to save me and take her life instead.

My doctors decided that the best treatment would be to add chemotherapy as well as a high dose of steroids to get my illness under control. This was in addition to the seven other pills I would have to take every day. Back then, using chemotherapy was experimental and they weren't sure how long it would take to get the best chance at remission. Because of that, I took chemo for two straight years. Let that sink in, two long years of chemo. The chemotherapy drug they used is called Cytoxan. I never liked the idea of pumping something through my veins that sounded like "toxin."

Cytoxan chemotherapy is still used today for severe Lupus; however, it is used in shorter bursts of treatment. I have never met anyone else who has taken it for two years straight like I did over 20 years ago. Back then, using Cytoxan chemotherapy was still in the research stage and they didn't know how long you needed to take it. So, in many ways, I became a human guinea pig.

I would joke with my doctors that I didn't feel that sick until they started trying to cure me. Sadly, many medical treatments feel worse than the disease they are designed to treat. For me, getting better meant feeling worse.

After my first year of chemotherapy treatments, I tried to negotiate the second year but they were having none of it. I had been raised in a family where you more or less did what your doctors said and that was the end of it.

Chemotherapy today is tough, and it was hard back then too. The first week I couldn't eat at all due to constant nausea and vomiting. Nothing would stay down. By the second week, the nausea was a bit better, but I was afraid to eat and have to vomit. By the third week, I started to come back, but I would still feel dizzy. Around the fourth week, I began to feel like myself again, and then went right back on to the next treatment and started the whole cycle all over again.

Everyone reacts differently when things feel out of control. For me, I found my control in studying, so that was what I did. Whenever I felt clear-headed, I would read my biology textbook or something to get through it and pass the time. I preferred to think of my illness on an intellectual level, wondering how the cells were reacting to the treatment. I ended up always being ahead of my class and many probably thought I was another nerd. Okay I was and still am a nerd, but many started to think of me as the Teacher's Pet, especially when a teacher would stop to ask me how I was feeling or ask if I need a water break (cringe). No one knew that I was sick except for my teachers, and that's how I wanted it. It was bad enough being a patient and having my family look at me with those sad eyes; I wanted everyone else to treat me like a normal person.

Although the treatments were scary and excruciating at times, the truth is those doctors saved my life. After two grueling years of chemo and endless number of pills, the kidney disease finally went into remission. Remission is a condition where your disease is stable, it is still there, but it is not getting worse, and the symptoms are minimal. In remission, I had the strength to move on to college and follow my dreams, although I had to guard myself closely. Thanks to the doctors who saved my life, I decided to go into medicine and became a doctor myself. I wanted to help people who came to me in the same way my doctors had helped me.

Western medicine is excellent at saving your life and stopping an illness from killing you. However, despite all our medical knowledge it can't stop the disease from progressing. Lupus is a particularly devious disease that way; your body becomes its own worst enemy. Your body is full of inflammation and your immune system becomes confused and dangerous. It can no longer differentiate between the dangerous infections it is supposed to attack, and your own organs. It is also progressive, meaning it will get worse over time and will attack other organs, and lead to other autoimmune diseases. It is a terrifying disease, for both patients and doctors. One of my clients for nutrition-based healing said her doctor told her, "It would be easier for me to help you if you had HIV than Lupus."

With my newly born remission, my doctors sternly warned me to avoid stress, always get enough sleep each night, and to avoid sunlight.

At the young age of eighteen, it felt like my entire life had been shut down. No staying up all night at sleepovers? No going to the beach? Would I have no life at all?

Then I received the news that made any possible remaining fairy tale image of a future disappear. All that chemotherapy probably damaged my ovaries. If I could even have children, I shouldn't, because of the severity of the disease. Having children is a huge risk for women with Lupus, and many die trying to have children. Not only had Lupus taken away the last two years of my childhood, but I may also now be robbed of my future!

While I did take my doctor's advice very seriously, I also knew I had to follow my heart and dreams. I knew my life had a purpose; I wanted to help others be happier and healthier. I also wanted to experience love and adventure. I was determined to have my life and I told myself, "I will have my life."

I didn't know how long I would have left, or even how sick I would get in the future, but I would make every day mean something and I was determined to fully live every day I had. I encourage you to say "I will have my life" out loud. It helps.

This is incredibly important to believe and fight for. If you let it, Lupus can rob you of your life and your dreams – so don't let it do so!

Life after My Illness, College, and Then Medical School

One week after my last chemotherapy treatment, I had packed up and moved into my college dorm at Carnegie Mellon University.

I loved every moment of college and felt an even greater sense of gratitude for any form of normalcy. I enjoyed being able to hang out with friends, for being able to learn, and even for studying. Every day I could get up out of my bed and move forward.

I remember while everyone else was complaining about homework, I was thinking, *I love homework. I love going to lecture. I can't wait to wake up at 7 and get to class.* Ok maybe that last part was an exaggeration, but the fact is, I was truly overjoyed to have normal problems. It was nice for me to be able to just have to go to class and study and not have to worry about the chemo.

When you have Lupus, or any chronic disease, nothing sounds better than a normal life, and you don't take any of those normal events and things for granted. If someone complained that they had five finals in one day, I would rejoice at it because it was a normal problem that college kids that aren't in the hospital get to deal with.

I had a social life and a whole group of friends who didn't know that I had Lupus!

Because I was in a new city at a new college, I got to be plain old Brooke instead of "Oh Poor Brooke." So many people I have talked to who have Lupus have said, "Man, I want to talk to my family about something else, *anything else*, you know?" Of course, we know that our family loves us and means well and that they want to support us. It's just sometimes we want to say, "Can't you just talk to me about how sad you are that *One Life to Live* went off the air?" For me that was sad because I had been watching that show with my grandma since I was a little girl. We need time to talk about things besides our illness to preserve our sense of ourselves and who we were before our diagnosis.

Although my disease was considered to be in remission, my lab tests were always positive for Lupus, and I still had the occasional problem arise. If I stayed up too late or overdid it on exercise or stress, I would get joint pain, migraines, or have days when I felt like I was walking and moving under water. There were days when all I could do was lie in bed because my body felt so heavy and slow. It's so important to listen to your body and rest on days like this. Pushing yourself when you feel like marrying your bed can make it worse or prolong the pain. When I was in college, I always rested when my body demanded it, something I couldn't do later on that contributed to my eventual relapse.

Despite the occasional bad day, I did really well overall in college. I graduated with honors with a bachelor's degree in Biology and a Minor in Creative Writing, and at a time when only 40 percent of applicants got accepted into medical school, I was accepted into my first choice: Temple University School of Medicine. My dream came true!

Despite living the dream, things got hairy pretty fast. While I could easily avoid sunlight while I was studying for about twelve hours a day, avoiding stress, and getting enough sleep, well, got difficult. These days there are laws that prevent medical students or residents from working more than 80 hours a week, or for more than 30 hours straight. Back when I was in medical school, however, there was no such law regulating our hours. One week during my medical school rotations, I calculated that I had worked a total of one hundred hours!

This type of stress and these work hours can be hard on anybody, but they caught up with me in an especially bad and dangerous way.

Relapse

Before Medical School, my Lupus blood tests had been positive for Lupus but stable for four years, and I was considered to be in remission, despite still getting arthritis, weakness, or migraines if I didn't sleep or I became stressed.

Medical School pushed me hard and I could no longer protect my sleep and accomplish everything required of me. I remember being so exhausted during my surgery rotation that I would get home after 6 p.m., have a snack, and pass out on the couch at around 7 p.m. while my roommate watched Jeopardy. At some point in the night, I would crawl up to my bed in the dark only to have my alarm wake me up at 4 a.m. Then it was time to change my scrubs, brush my teeth, grab an apple, and get back to the hospital to do my pre-rounds on patients before my supervising resident got there.

By the time I did my family practice rotation in November 2003, I had started having episodes of double vision. Once or twice a day, I would feel a bit light-headed and unsteady, and then the entire world would be double, two identical images side by side. I would hold the wall and wait for what felt like 30 seconds to a minute, and then it would clear up again. I also noticed that I was getting red spots on my nails.

Being a diligent medical student, I went to my attending physician in family medicine and told her that I had Lupus and was now getting double vision and red spots on my nails. I asked her what she thought I should do. I don't think she was listening to me very closely because she told me it was probably nothing serious and went on with her day. I had a very bad feeling that she was wrong, but I decided to wait for Thanksgiving break to see my own doctors to getter a better evaluation. Before I had the chance, things got worse.

One day I had an especially dangerous and frightening episode that thankfully did not leave me or anyone else hurt. I was working in the family clinic giving tuberculosis tests and flu shots like a typical medical student when I suddenly felt very confused and disoriented. I couldn't tell if I was awake or dreaming. Memories of the day passed through my mind, but they felt distant and surreal. I wasn't even sure if I had really treated any patients that day, it was like a dream. I couldn't talk or move. I must have passed out because I woke up to find myself collapsed at my desk with my head on a chart. The office had closed, and nobody was there. The doctors and residents had all left me there.

I suppose they thought I was another overworked and exhausted medical student like the many that they had seen before I came onto the scene. They may have even thought I was catching up on sleep on the job. When I look back now, it is truly terrifying. I could have died.

After an unknown amount of time, I was finally able to get myself up and to my car. I truly do not know how this happened, but I was able to drive myself home. I couldn't remember any of the streets, and it all looked so unfamiliar to me. I was scared, but all I could think about was getting home. Have you ever had your body drive you home while your brain was otherwise distracted? Somehow, my body knew how to get me back to my apartment, and I somehow made it home without hurting myself or anyone else in the process.

I crawled into my bed and slept for a few hours. When I woke up, I felt back to normal and met up with some doctor friends I had made plans with. I told them about my episode, and they laughed it off saying I needed more sleep. I knew, however, something was seriously wrong with me and I was terrified to find out what it was.

When I got back home for Thanksgiving vacation, I went right to my doctors. They were extremely concerned, and I was immediately sent in to get a CT scan, MRIs, and a bunch of blood tests. My doctors were like family at this point, and they couldn't hide the worry in their eyes.

When the tests came back, it was time to face the bad news. I had developed a new autoimmune disease. This time I was making antibodies to my clotting blood cells, it was called anticardiolipin antibody. This was causing me to create blood clots that were spreading all over my body. The clots were getting stuck in the small vessels in my fingernails causing the red spots known as splinter hemorrhages. The blood clots were also going to my brain causing the double vision and the episode I had at the clinic, which I now understood as a transient ischemic attack – a ministroke that thankfully did not cause permanent damage.

I was at high risk of a serious stroke or pulmonary embolism, and I was put on injectable blood thinners. I had to inject myself in the stomach or backside with a needle every day. I was told I had to do this for the rest of my life or risk having a stroke or pulmonary embolism, which could kill me or leave me permanently disabled.

The blood thinners, while they worked, left me covered in bruises from the injections and even the most unnoticed papercut would cause an embarrassing rush of blood that would quickly cover my hands in blood. On blood thinners, you take much longer to make scabs and the blood keeps flowing. I also knew that an accident or bump to the head could be life-threatening – I could bleed out of a wound or bleed into my brain. These medications are serious.

With the help of the medicine, the double vision stopped, and the blood clots were dissolved. Once again, modern medicine had saved my life, but it was not giving me health.

Living with the thought of "what next?" hanging over you is frightening if you let it sink in. What I learned in medical school was that with Lupus, I was more susceptible to getting almost any other disease there is. Lupus is considered to be chronic and debilitating. This means that the condition should stay with me throughout my life, and it should get worse over time. I knew and dreaded the fact that things would only get worse as I got older.

To make things worse, I had been told that the chemotherapy that I had endured not only put me at a higher risk for cancer, but it may have damaged my ovaries, which could prevent me from being able to have children. I had already been warned that pregnancy was dangerous if you had Lupus and kidney failure; many women have died trying to have children with this disease. Now that I had the blood clot antibody, I was informed that it was almost certainly a death wish to attempt a pregnancy. All women are more vulnerable to blood clots when they are pregnant, but I was already high risk without the added clotting risk from pregnancy hormones. Now, not only could pregnancy cause a Lupus flare-up that could hurt me or the unborn baby, but it was also highly probable that a blood clot would kill me or leave me with a paralyzing stroke.

Again, I mourned for my fragile health. I cried for about two weeks, especially over the fact I would need to take injections for the rest of my life. I was finally so close to my dream of being a doctor, and once again, I almost died while my body attacked itself mercilessly. Once again, I was a patient on dangerous drugs. I had almost lost the one organ I counted on the most, my brain – the very organ that helped me survive kidney failure had been under attack.

After I had allowed myself my period of mourning, I took a deep breath, accepted it, and allowed myself to feel gratitude. I was still here! Once again, I had beaten the odds because of my incredible doctors and the fact that at the very least, there was medicine to save me.

Western medicine once again saved my life. If it weren't for modern medicine, I would have died at 16 from kidney failure or of a stroke at the age of 24.

I still honor and value what medications and modern medicine can do for us. However, I also know their limitations. They could save my life but could not give me my health.

Despite the pitfalls and challenges that I knew were before me, I was determined to continue pushing onward, pursue my dreams, and follow my heart. I was close to graduating medical school and so close to achieving my goals. Once again, I was told to "take it easy" and to "avoid stress." I said, "I will have my life."

Falling in Love and Other Miracles

It was March 2004, and I was two months away from graduating medical school. I was stable on my medication and feeling much better. Not only was I within months of receiving my M.D., but I had also matched for my first choice for my residency program, at Harbor-UCLA Medical Center. It combined the UCLA education I admired with full immersion into their community hospital where I would be learning from and treating the poor and underserved, which was a great desire in my heart. Often the poor get subpar medical care, but here at this enormous teaching hospital, there were good doctors, medical students and residents all trying their best to help them.

While I reveled in the countdown before graduation, I was enjoying my final moments in Pittsburgh, where I had completed my medical school rotations. I was purely going out to have fun and mingle. My heart was so full from my personal sense of accomplishment and my excitement for my move to sunny California and starting my residency program that I just wanted to enjoy my friends and go out to have fun. While I was happy to accept invitations to go out on dates, I was not interested in anything too serious; I was way too happy and fulfilled being single. Meeting my future husband was as far from my mind as it could be.

Yet that is when I met the most amazing man I could ever meet. He is a brilliant scientist, a true intellectual, who also happened to be sensitive, sweet, open-minded, openhearted, and gorgeous. He challenged me, made me laugh, and made me tingle every time he looked my way. His name is Thomas Tadlock.

We fell in love so quickly it was overwhelming and beautiful. We would stay up all night and lay in each other's arms as we talked about our future and our dreams. Together we would cry uncontrollable happy tears until the sunrise rose through the high windows in his Pittsburgh loft.

A month into our relationship, Thomas told me he wanted to get married. How desperately I wanted to say "yes!" I truly did, I wanted nothing more than to say that little three-letter word.

Yet, I had not told him about my disease because I felt it was too early in the relationship. I also didn't want to bring up such a depressing topic. Privately, I was scared he would turn and run away to save himself the sight of watching me grow weak and disabled as time passed. Would he even want to marry a woman who could never have children? A woman who would eventually need to be taken care of? A woman who would die far too young?

Still, he deserved to know. He had to know. Tearfully, I choked on my words as they tumbled out. I told him about my disease, my inability to have children, the fact he would end up taking care of me, and perhaps the worst of all, I may be disabled from arthritis and organ disease by my thirties.

Certainly not a romantic topic to discuss following a proposal!

When I looked up at him, I saw his handsome and sad face. Tears were running down his cheeks and he was frozen.

Seconds ticked by that felt like an eternity.

Until my dying day, I will never forget the look in his eyes when he took my hand and said, "I would rather spend a little time with you, than a lifetime with anyone else."

At that moment, I felt more joy and hope than I knew was possible! This man wanted to love me for as long as he could!

I had never before dreamed of a white dress, only a white coat, and suddenly I was planning a wedding!

I left for California only a month later, just two months after we had met, and I excitedly found a small apartment for the two of us. Now I just had to wait for Thomas to get his business and home managed so he could move to California himself and we could start our life together.

I knew nothing about California as I had grown up in the Northeast all my life. It was quite the culture shock to see just how expensive living there was compared to the prices in Pittsburgh! To put things into perspective I had been living in a three-story house in Pittsburgh that was completely renovated, and I paid $695 a month for it. I couldn't even find a studio apartment in LA for that price!

I started to look into an area called Long Beach, which was about 45 minutes away from the hospital but more affordable. I had no idea that at the time that there were many gang-filled neighborhoods in that area, but I did wonder why it was so much more affordable.

I had found one listing called "Zen Loft at the Ocean," which was located on Naples Island. I saw on a map that it was indeed surrounded by the ocean and was its own little paradise. It was also a straight shot to the highway that would take me to the hospital. It turned out to be a renovated motel, and the "Zen loft" was a lofted bed over a living space the size of a small room. There was a dorm refrigerator and a hot plate for cooking. It was barely enough room for me to live on my own, and definitely too small for my two large cats and my hunky fiancée! Disappointed, I asked the manager if they had any larger rooms. He said they had one downstairs that was a double; it was converted from the original office of the motel. It had two tiny rooms: a bedroom/bathroom and a kitchen/living room. It was still tiny, but it had a full-sized stove and a refrigerator – and for $1150 a month, it included utilities. As I stood in the tiny apartment, I could smell and feel the ocean breeze and my decision was made. This would be our first home in California.

It wasn't easy living in paradise, though! I was completely broke! Most people don't realize that doctors start out making less per hour than the average waiter. I had been a student until the age of 27 and started out as an intern barely making $600 a week. Between rent, my student loan payments, and meager groceries, I was constantly at zero balance (or overdrawn) in my bank account. I couldn't even afford the rent without Thomas' help.

When I first flew out to California, Thomas took a few days off to help me move. When we first moved me into our tiny apartment, I couldn't even afford furniture. I got a free coffee table off Craigslist, a chair from a neighbor, and then spent the first couple of weeks sleeping on the bedroom floor with nothing but a pillow and blanket a friend had given me. None of this troubled me emotionally at all though – I was on cloud nine! I was about to start my residency training – my dream job – and I was loved by the most amazing person I had ever met. On the first night I spent in the apartment, I remember lying on the floor with Thomas beside me. I could not stop thinking about how joyful and grateful I was. I told him, "No matter how much money we might make or how successful we might become, I never want to forget that lying here on the floor of this tiny little apartment, I am the happiest I have ever been." And I was.

Sadly, Thomas was not able to move in with me right away, and he soon had to pull himself from my arms and board the plane back to Pittsburgh. He had his own business and owned a condo in Pittsburgh. His life was there. Right before we met, he had bought a fixer-upper loft. He had been planning to turn it into a stylish modern space but had been working on it slowly up until that point. He committed to finishing his renovations on his condo so he could find a tenant or a buyer, and decided to find someone to manage his business as soon as possible so he could move to California, and we could start our lives together. After spending two dreamy months together, Thomas and I would live on opposite ends of the country for the next six months.

We spent every possible moment on the phone. Thomas even changed his phone plan to mine so we could have unlimited minutes after his first phone bill made his jaw drop.

We didn't have bluetooth or hands-free back then, so we walked around with our mobile phones in our pockets with the wired earpieces going up into our ears. I'd call him the moment I finished up at the hospital and we would just keep the phones connected until we fell asleep. Sometimes we wouldn't talk, we would simply be going about our day, him working on his loft, me at the video store or the supermarket, just feeling better having any connection to each other. It might sound a little crazy, but it really felt like we were still spending our time together in spite of the distance. I remember going to Blockbuster to get a video a year later, and the cashier said she honestly didn't recognize me at first because I didn't have my earpiece in!

While I endured the grueling schedule of an intern, Thomas worked nonstop on his condo and his business. He also booked flights to California for every weekend he could get away. There was never a question in either of our minds that we were meant to be together, and he showed me his devotion every day.

Six months later, he finished up the renovations on his condo, turning it into the stylish New York-style loft that he always dreamed of living in. He spent one night in his fancy new loft and the next morning he handed over the keys to the new owner and left for California with only his car and whatever fit in his backseat and trunk, where he would move into the tiny apartment with two big cats and me. I always joke that he pulled a *Good Will Hunting* and "went to see about a girl!" He drove across the country, only stopping once to sleep for four hours before showing up at my door. We talked excitedly on the phone during his journey, counting the minutes until he would get there. When he showed up at my door, we both pulled out our earpieces and embraced passionately before he passed out on our bed for two days straight to recover from his six months of manic renovating and sleep-deprived driving.

Thomas and I had decided on an extremely small ceremony in Maui. There were only twelve guests, our parents, his sister, my grandparents, and our very best friends. We agreed to a small wedding for two important reasons: one, we didn't want it to be a stressful event, or one spent trying to say hello to cousins and other people who were practically strangers to us. You know the type of cousins that you only ever see at weddings or other major family events but whom you barely know. We wanted it to be a celebration of our love that we would enjoy to the fullest, with the people who loved us most. I feel Thomas said it best, "I only want people at our wedding who will cry."

There was also another very large benefit to marrying Thomas Tadlock. Some of you may be familiar with his name. He is very well-known in the fitness industry for being the No. 1 rapid fat loss expert in the country and perhaps even the world. When I met him, he had recently been featured on MTV as "the hottest body at the beach house" and was hired by MTV to personally train recording artists that might have a beer belly and need to have hot abs in their music video only a few weeks down the road, and he could do it!

Thomas had figured out that if you nourish your cells at a biochemical level, they can dramatically improve in function and cause a surge of health and a super-fast metabolism. Follow the guide, do some exercise, and the fat should melt right off!

I was no longer that skinny girl from the days when I was a teenager. Before meeting Thomas, whenever I wanted to lose weight, I did what I'd learned in medical school and from every other woman I'd ever met: restrict calories and exercise. At the time I met him, I was about a size 7/8, eating small meals, and exercising two hours a day. When we fell in love, I started skipping the gym to hang out with him more and found myself eating everything in sight! I always joke that falling in love makes you feel invincible – like even calories can't hurt you! I remember thinking it was so romantic that Thomas would feed me ice cream in bed. Who was I to turn that down? Understandably, the pounds started to pack on.

When I moved to California and started my residency, I didn't have access to my old gym and spent my limited free time sleeping. I was eating the ironically unhealthy cafeteria food served to me at the hospital, and that combination of poor food and lack of exercise led to some more extra pounds. By the time Thomas moved in with me, I was a size 10/11 and not too happy about it. I suppose it's something a lot of us women do, we get thin to attract them, they love us when we get a little bit pudgy, and then we race to get thin again for the wedding!

So, like every bride, I wanted to look my best at our wedding. There was the added pressure of getting married in Maui, and all the photographs we would be taking in swimsuits. I told Thomas I wanted his help "getting hot" for our wedding. I didn't want to stress out my body with severe restrictions. I also needed my energy for my job as an intern and couldn't deal with low blood sugar and do my best at my job. I definitely did not want to deal with the inevitable bad moods that coming with skipping meals. I had many girlfriends who had starved themselves for their weddings. They were miserable leading up to the big day, and then gained weight rapidly when they started eating again after the wedding. One of my friends starved herself skinny for her wedding, and then gained 20 pounds on her honeymoon!

Thomas created a plan for me to get fit as quickly as possible while taking the best care of my body. He named it *The Dream Body Program* because it was designed to get me my dream body. He had me eating all day long and exercising an hour a day. When I first saw how much he wanted me to eat, I was afraid I would gain weight – it was much more than I was used to eating. He joked with me that doctors are the most difficult clients because we think we know everything. I sheepishly accepted his chiding and agreed to do it his way. I did his plan and stuck to it. Four months later, I had gone from a size eleven to a size three and the results have been permanent!

The weight loss alone was a great thing, but I soon discovered more added benefits I had not considered or yet realized. I was now feeling better, even amazing. I felt energetic and strong. I could work my 30-hour shifts at the hospital without getting migraines and arthritis. In fact, the aches and pains had completely gone away! I decided to continue eating that way so I could continue to feel great and healthy.

When it came time to have my routine blood work a couple of weeks before our wedding, we had amazing results that no one could have ever predicted. My Lupus titers were undetectable, ANA was negative, DS DNA was undetectable, complement levels were normal. All indicators for Lupus were gone as if I never had the disease at all! The clotting antibodies, Anticardiolipin AB, were only mildly elevated, and would not be considered treatable if it weren't for my history of blood clots.

Could my results have really been this good? Perhaps my work got mixed up with someone else's or someone, somewhere, had goofed and was due for quite the yelling at.

My doctor could not explain it, recommending that I go enjoy my wedding and come back to retest my labs when I got back. The test was repeated the next month and ALL of my tests were completely normal. Even the Anticardiolipin AB test was normal. They couldn't see any sign of the disease at all.

The doctors couldn't explain it. Diseases like mine don't magically disappear. Even in remission, all of the indicators for Lupus are readily observable on blood tests. According to my blood work, I didn't have a disease.

My doctors decided to continue my lab tests every 3-4 months as before and my results only got better. My high cholesterol that I had been told was "just bad genetics" was now perfect. My heart rate and blood pressure were at levels you normally only see in marathon runners, and I was far from such an athlete. My body felt strong and energetic, and I no longer felt like a sick person.

After a year of feeling amazing and having normal blood work, I was ready to move on with my life. I asked my doctor why I was still taking medication after a year of perfect blood tests. It appeared as if we were both just treating our anxiety about what would happen to me without medication, rather than treating my tests results and my clinical presentation. I especially wanted to go off my blood thinner medication. If I didn't need it anymore, why should I take it? It was hard work convincing my doctor and my family to approve of this idea, which seemed so incredibly radical and potentially dangerous. Everyone was terrified I would have a stroke. I did vow to return quickly to my doctor's care if I experienced any symptoms. After living with Lupus for 16 years, I knew my own body extremely well. I didn't want to take any chances with my health or my life, but I also didn't want to take unnecessary medications that had serious side effects of their own. Incredibly, it has now been 10 years since I've had any symptoms of Lupus and my blood work remains a reflection of my good health.

After enjoying over two years of health, getting stronger every day, enjoying things that I was told I could never do, like taking a cruise through the Panama Canal out in the hot sun all day long every day, dancing late into the night with my husband, and completing my four-year residency and graduating as a Board-Certified Medical Doctor, I decided I was ready to embrace even more of the life that I was once told I could never have. I mentioned earlier that the doctors warned me not to have children. I wanted to revisit that issue considering my newfound health that I had proven I could not only sustain but also continue to enhance over two years.

I had started dreaming about having a baby. In my dreams, I could see my baby so clearly, and I would hold him in my arms and feel his warmth against me. Then I would wake up sad and feeling his loss. My body was telling me I was ready; I could feel it through and through. Convincing my husband was another matter altogether.

Thomas felt like we had been given this amazing gift; instead of preparing himself to take care of me as my body failed organ by organ, and burying me far too young, he was now looking forward to many more happy years together. Having a baby could be risking it all. I felt strongly that I was no longer sick, and that my body was ready. I knew my body well, and it was not the same one that had been sick for so long: not only did I feel it, but also the blood tests continued to confirm it.

Next, I had to break it to my best friends and closest family. The idea of me getting pregnant horrified my parents and worried my best friend who had long ago volunteered to be my surrogate if I ever decided I wanted children. My mother also stepped forward and volunteered to be a surrogate. I am very lucky to be so loved and guarded by my loved ones. I gently explained that I was going to do it, that I had no desire to risk my life, that I truly believed that I could carry a baby safely.

My husband and I set ourselves to the fun work of creating a baby, and we finally were successful! After a day of bloating and vomiting, I got a pregnancy test and tested positive. Then I bought five more pregnancy tests because I just couldn't believe it, and they were positive too! I texted my mother a photograph of the 6 positive tests and she nervously texted back that maybe I should take another one!

When I met my new obstetrician, she was immediately gravely concerned about my medical history. I don't think she really heard me or even believed me when I told her that I had been healthy and Lupus-free for three years. She thought I was going to ruin a long remission. She echoed the warnings I had heard years ago that pregnancy could trigger my immune system and cause a raging relapse of Lupus.

Since I was considered "high risk" because of my medical history, she sent me to a high-risk OB specialist. The high-risk OB looked over my body, labs, ultrasounds, and said I was one of the healthiest pregnant moms she had seen and did not consider me high risk at the time. She sent me back to my regular obstetrician. While my OB was wary, she agreed to see me through the pregnancy. Just to be safe, she monitored me with monthly ultrasounds, which I did not mind. I was happy to see my baby once a month!

I had been warned that my Lupus could return, triggered by my pregnancy, and my immune system could restart with full force. That never happened. I was warned about the risk of blood clots, but my blood remained healthy. While I was very nauseous thanks to those healthy high levels of hormones, my immune system functioned perfectly well. My little baby grew healthy and strong inside my belly.

Forty weeks later, I delivered a healthy baby boy, Solomon, named for my favorite grandfather. Solomon was breech, butt first, and so I needed a cesarean section to deliver him. The surgery went well, and I was up and about the same day as the surgery. The second set of warnings had come in from the doctors, that giving birth causes the immune system to come back online powerfully after the more immunosuppressed state of pregnancy, and I was now, post-partum, at the highest risk for relapse of Lupus. It never happened. Not only was my baby boy perfectly healthy, but I was also in great shape too! I felt very little pain at all from the surgery and felt strong and energetic, ready to go home. My blood tests remained perfectly normal.

Not only that, but thanks to the health of my cells, I had a super-fast metabolism, meaning my body could adapt to different states quickly, and recover quickly.

While I gained a healthy 40lbs during my first pregnancy, I was back in my size 3 jeans nine days after I gave birth, without doing anything but cuddling and nursing my baby and eating a lot to compensate for that intense hunger that breastfeeding a baby brings!

Two years ago, I brought my second son, Alexander, into the world. He was born healthy and strong. Nobody worried about my pregnancy that time around. Everyone, including my doctors, knew that I was healthy and nothing was going to go wrong.

My obstetrician is a firm believer in the safety of a repeat cesarean section after your first one. I was tempted to try a vaginal birth just to flex my female powers, but my beloved doctor was very much against it after having a recent patient rupture during an attempted VBAC, landing her and the baby in the ICU. My husband pleaded with me to "just do everything the same way as before," and I agreed.

Once again, the surgery was easy to recover from. When my OB came in to check on me later that day, I complimented her. "You are an amazing surgeon!" because I recovered so quickly after hearing many women lament in person and online over how difficult the recovery is from a c-section.

She responded, "I am a great surgeon, but you have an amazing ability to heal."

Her words still astound me when I think about them.

You have an amazing ability to heal.

Me, the same woman who became sick at 16 years old. The same woman who has almost died from kidney failure and blood clots. The same woman who used to spend weeks in bed trying to recover from a little cold that a friend walked around with for a few days. The same woman who still has a scar from a giant abscess that formed on my hip when I was eighteen, because my body couldn't even heal a pimple.

Now, at thirty-eight years old, now I have an amazing ability to heal. And it's all because I made some simple changes in my diet.

Many doctors who meet me now find it hard to believe that I have ever had Lupus, but one look at my old charts, or conversation with my old doctor, and there is no question that not only was I sick, but my disease was also aggressive and life-threatening.

I do not consider myself to be "in remission" anymore but rather, I do not have a disease.

The Healing Nutrition Plan: 6 Easy Steps To Healing With Supermarket Foods

It's important to realize this is not just a nutrition plan; it is a lifestyle change. This is about learning how to truly eat to live, to heal, and to feel the very best you possibly can.

When going through this nutrition plan you are feeding your body the very best foods to nourish your cells and allow them to do the work they need to do to decrease inflammation and heal. In spite of this, it is very possible that you may feel lousy due to released toxins and withdrawal symptoms as your body detoxifies itself. Clients have reported anything from tiredness and headaches to rashes as their bodies cleansed and detoxified. This process is important and, once it passes, you will feel better than you ever thought possible. It is very important for your body to detoxify itself so it can become healthy again. If you want to minimize detox, add the green smoothies and raw foods to your usual diet 1-2 weeks before you complete the rest of the changes to your diet. If the symptoms are unbearable, you can take it slowly, making one change at a time, and only making the next change when you feel ready. For example, you can keep eating your usual diet, and add green smoothies. Then stop dairy products, etc., until you have completed the transformation of your eating to a low-inflammation lifestyle. This usually bypasses the detox process, although it slows down the results. The important thing is that you get there, and you must decide the path you need to take. Choose the path that you believe will ensure your success.

It is also very important that you do not starve yourself! If you are hungry, then you should eat something healthy. This is a plan to make sure your body becomes super nourished so it can heal at a cellular level. When you eat this way, you can trust your hunger and eat unlimited amounts of the recommended food because your body is asking for more nourishment. Never let yourself go hungry. If you feel hungry, go for a green smoothie, some fresh veggies, fruits, or a handful of raw nuts. Always keep something with you so you don't end up hungry or tempted to go off this nutrition plan. If you are in a bind, you can always stop at a market for some fresh fruit, grab a salad or go to a place where they make fresh juices or smoothies to hold you over.

Step 1:
Eliminate Animal Products

Animal Products include all types of meat like beef, pork, lamb, fish, and chicken. It also includes eggs and dairy products. The reason these foods must be avoided at all costs is because they cause massive amounts of inflammation in the body.

Inflammation is normally the body's healthy response to injury. However, when the inflammation becomes chronic, or continuous, such as due to constant assault on the gut by the wrong foods, the inflammation becomes the cause of destructive diseases, like Lupus, Scleroderma, Rheumatoid Arthritis, Colitis, and many other chronic inflammatory diseases. Research has indicated animal-derived products are inflammatory in multiple different ways. A recent study in *Scientific American* showed that when the gut is exposed to saturated fat, it causes the destruction of the healthy protective bacteria in the gut, which then leads to inflammation of the gut wall, initiation of an immune response, which leads to tissue damage and even hemorrhage.[1]

Meat and dairy also are a direct source of arachidonic acid and omega-6 fatty acids, both of which directly produce inflammatory immune mediators, prostaglandins, and leukotrienes, which go right to work creating inflammation in the body. The more meat and dairy you consume, the more inflammation you create.

One study published in the *American Journal of Epidemiology* did a meta-analysis of 9 prospective studies that showed that eating animal products increases the risk of all-cause mortality, meaning it raises your risk of dying from any disease.[3] Most folks are familiar with the idea that eating meat increases their risk of heart disease, but don't realize that eating meat increases their risk of death from all causes.

Our society consumes enormous amounts of dairy products in milk, cheese, yogurts, and ice cream. This includes milk, yogurt, and cheeses.

Cheese was the hardest one for me to give up! I really did not want to cut it out of my life, but when I read the research on how toxic dairy is for the body, I knew it had to go. Dairy not only causes massive amounts of inflammation, but it has also been shown by Dr. T. Colin Campbell to be a cancer promoter on the DNA level – which means it gives the DNA the signal to create cancer![2] Other studies have supported the link between prostate cancer and other cancers like colon cancer and the consumption of animal products.[4,5] Dairy foods also increase growth hormones, which cause cancer. Studies have shown that dairy increases Insulin-like Growth Factor, IGF-1, which promotes cancer growth and accelerated aging.[7] IGF-1 is one of the most powerful promoters of cancer growth ever discovered for cancers of the breast, prostate, lung, and colon.[6] Dairy products also raise your estrogen levels, since the milk is being generated by a dairy cow that is either pregnant or just gave birth, since like us, cows only lactate when they have offspring. The practice of continuously milking cows throughout pregnancy has been shown to raise estrogen levels, which are known risk factors for breast, uterus, and prostate cancer.[8,9]

When I teach this information to my clients, their first concern is, "how do I get my calcium?" They are worried that giving up dairy products might cause osteoporosis, an idea that comes straight from dairy industry propaganda and commercials. What science has shown is that dairy products have actually cause bone loss, explaining why countries that have the highest rates of dairy consumption like the USA, Canada, Norway, Sweden, Australia, and New Zealand, also have the highest rates of osteoporosis.[10,11] The lowest rates are among people who eat the fewest animal-derived foods like natives of rural Asia and rural Africa. [10,11] These people also have lower calcium intake overall than we do.

Calcium is abundant and easy to absorb from green leafy vegetables like kale and broccoli, without the risks that come with consuming dairy products.

Dairy is also especially bad for children. Not only does milk and other dairy products set them up for bone loss and cancer, it's been shown to be the most likely trigger for Type I Diabetes, also known as Insulin-Dependant Diabetes.[12, 13] In children with a genetic predisposition to Type I diabetes, exposure to milk has been shown to directly increase the development of the disease in the infant with early exposure. [12, 13] The theory is that the baby's immature immune system may create antibodies to milk protein, which it later confuses with the pancreas, creating an autoimmune attack that ultimately destroys the pancreas and creates lifelong illness and disability.

When I read this research, I sat on my couch and cried, thinking about how many children were suffering because their doctors are telling mothers to give cow milk to their young children, essentially poisoning them. As doctors, we swear to first "do no harm," but in this scenario, doctors are causing a lot of harm. I thought to myself, there must be some scientific data that supports the idea of giving toddlers milk since it was drummed into my head in medical school that everything we do must be "evidence-based." Sadly, I could not find one article that supported this archaic practice, so I assume it is based on an old habit being passed down from doctor to resident without being questioned. The data is now overwhelming that dairy is toxic to humans, and as physicians, we need to do better.

There is life after dairy, and when I finally did give up cheese and dairy ice cream, to my surprise, I did not really miss it.

I have had many patients tell me that as addicted to cheese as they were before they started, they felt much better when they remove dairy from their diet. There are also many alternatives to dairy these days that can taste quite pleasant. These include milks and yogurts made from almonds and coconuts. These can often be found at your local grocery store and for a decent price.

Step 2:
Eliminate Added Oils

In step 1, I already discussed the dangers of saturated fat from meat and dairy products. Omega-6 fatty acids can also be found in high levels of vegetable oils so they must also be avoided.

Omega-6 fatty acids are essential for the body and must be consumed since your body cannot create them. The issue is that most foods people eat nowadays, such as meat, vegetable oils, and processed foods, are laden with omega-6 fatty acids, but their balancing counterpart, omega-3s are largely absent. The problem in this is that omega-6 fatty acids are used by the body to create inflammatory immune cells. Conversely, omega-3s are responsible for creating the anti-inflammatory immune cells. The result is that most people are suffering from massive amounts of chronic inflammation, which leads to chronic diseases.

One of the fastest ways to minimize inflammation and jump-start the healing process is to eliminate the excess sources of omega-6 fatty acids. As I mentioned earlier, animal products are a source of omega-6 fatty acids. Even more so are all of the vegetable oils, with the exception of olive oil.

Examine the table below and you can quickly see how both animal products like meat and eggs and oils both lead the production of Arachidonic Acid, which is then converted into inflammatory immune cells, which create inflammation. If you want to dramatically and rapidly reduce the inflammation, and therefore inflammatory illness, you need to eliminate these main causes of inflammation.

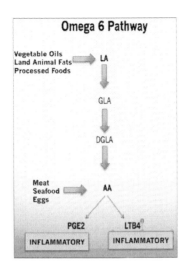

The flooding of our bodies with these omega-6 fatty acids just drives the body to create more and more inflammation, which creates more illness and impairs your body's ability to heal.

When you think about it, it would be entirely impossible to obtain the amount of oils you get in a serving of soybean oil by simply eating soybeans. For this reason, some specialists consider all oils to be processed foods, even though there are no additives, because the soybeans, olives, etc. must go through the extraction process to obtain the oils.

I've had a handful of clients who came to me for chronic issues who were already vegan and were perplexed at their remaining symptoms. The continued eating of processed foods and vegetable oils is usually the culprit, and when we correct their omega-6 to omega-3 ratio, they feel better quickly.

I did mention that olive oil is not a big source of omega-6, so if you need a bit of oil to sauté your vegetables, that's the one to use. However, don't overdo it, because too much of any oil will disturb the fluidity of your blood in your blood vessels and the responsiveness of your cells to the signals they need to receive. [14] It basically gums up the system while it's in your body. Oils, even olive oil, raise blood triglycerides (fats) immediately after eating them and decreased the function of the precious lining of the blood vessels.[14]

If you want to use some olive oil, I suggest getting a spray bottle and spraying the pan with a couple squirts to keep it nonstick.

I highly recommend that you investigate the numerous cooking methods available for oil-free cooking by simply using Google to search for "oil free cooking recipes." You may be amazing at how well sautéed vegetables come out when you use some water or vegetable broth instead of oil.

Now, when I talk about avoiding added fats, I am not talking about avoiding whole plant foods that are fatty, like avocados and coconuts. I have seen many well-meaning health coaches misinterpret the toxicity of oils to mean that people should limit these foods, which results in very sad clients! I had a friend once tell me she avoids avocados because:

"I can't bear to eat only half and put it away, so I just don't eat them!"

Perplexed, I asked, "why not eat the whole thing?" And she cried back,

"because of the faaaaaat!"

I tried to reassure her that the fat in a whole avocado would not slow down her weight-loss and fitness goals, but it was a hard sell. She had heard too many "experts" tell her the opposite.

Understand that fat in whole foods is easily recognized and processed by the body. I myself eat 2-3 avocados a day most days; they are filling, creamy, and delicious! When I was in the process of transforming my health and losing all that weight, I was using guacamole as my primary method of getting my raw veggies down; I could only eat a few pieces of plain raw broccoli on its own, but put a cup of guacamole dip in front of me and I could eat the entire head of broccoli! So don't worry about the fat content in fresh whole plant foods, just avoid adding oils and fats to your food. Fats from whole foods are an important part of your diet for healthy cells, especially flax and chia seeds which I will explain more in Step 5.

The more you avoid added oils, the better your cells, organs, and immune system will function, and the faster you will heal.

Step 3:
Eliminate Processed Foods

Processed foods are products that you can buy that contain ingredients that do not occur in nature. People call them foods, but they're more like synthesized food-like products. So what exactly are processed foods? One quick way to find out is to grab a can or box from your kitchen and read the label. If it has a long list of ingredients that you cannot pronounce or it cannot be produced without a lab, it is processed.

Pick up an apple and check out the ingredients. Apple. Not processed and pretty simple, right?

The Food and Drug Administration didn't actually start requiring companies to even label foods with additives until the 1950s, and then later in the 1960s with ingredients. In the 1950s, the American Diet had taken a turn for the worse: processed foods became mass distributed with the big new highways and were made more popular by television ads. Housewives were urged to take a break and serve ready-to-eat pre-made frozen meals and use of food additives exploded.

To this day, it is normal in many households to reach for a box or a can when preparing a meal or to grab something from the freezer and stick it in the microwave. Eating this way is convenient, and often cheap, but it does not provide any nourishment to the body. That is the real reason we are supposed to eat, to nourish ourselves.

Processed foods are not only lacking in nourishment, they have been shown to cause inflammation in the body shortly after consuming them.[15] This includes processed sugars as well as refined grains such as processed breads, cereals, pizzas, and tortillas, which have been shown to increase inflammation markers in the bloodstream and directly increase rates of diabetes and heart disease.[16] One of the primary ways processed foods increase inflammation is because they are loaded with inflammatory oils high in omega 6 that you learned about in step 2.

When you are trying to heal your body, all foods that increase inflammation must be avoided.

If you can eliminate animal products, excess oils, and processed foods from your diet, then you will immediately cause a decrease in the inflammation in your body, and you will start feeling better very quickly. If the idea of getting rid of all three at once is a bit intimidating, start with step 1 and work your way down. This doesn't have to be a race to the finish line, do it in a way that you know will be sustainable to you. If you start with just those the items mentioned in steps 1, 2 and 3, then you are getting a good head start on improving your health. Our bodies were not and are not meant to digest any of these foods – yet they have become the main sources of food for many people today. That is why people are so sick. If you are one of those people who eat mainly meat, dairy, oils, and processed foods, then take this as good news, because there is hope! The body can recover if you get out of its way by stopping the constant assault on it with these dangerous foods. You can make a difference in your health just by changing your shopping list.

After having eliminated all of the foods that can cause illness, you may be asking yourself, "Now what?" Now you need to fill your body with the foods that heal you.

Step 4:
Hyper-Nourish Yourself with Raw Plant Foods.

Did you know that all of the original medication came from the rainforest? Our original medicine came from plants! Once scientists figured out how to synthesize these medicines, the pharmaceutical company started making them and made a fortune and they still do. While I see the value of prescription medications, which can be lifesaving, we must not ignore the natural health-giving medicines that grow on the earth! We don't need to go to the rainforest to get our medicine, we can go to the supermarket!

In the United States of America, the most commonly eaten fruit or vegetable is ketchup, followed by fried potatoes! That means that even though many Americans are obese, they are in fact extremely malnourished.

Put together all of the things I've talked about so far, you can understand how we have become so sick! We are eating a huge array of inflammatory foods like meat, dairy, processed foods, and oils, *and* we are not getting any of the vital nutrients we need for health or healing, by eating such a sparse amount of necessary plant foods. This sounds like a recipe for disaster, and indeed, it has been.

For many clients who are nervous about giving up the foods they are used to, I have them start here, by adding what they are missing. What I have discovered is that even if people continue eating the unhealthy foods, adding the nourishing foods will create impressive improvements in their health. While complete healing does not occur until they put all the steps into place, this usually gives people the encouragement and motivation to start doing more for themselves because they see the power of foods. They also feel so much better, they are eager to find out how to get even more results.

If you are hesitant or nervous about giving up your typical foods all at once, I encourage you to start here. If you are going to eat harmful foods, at least start adding the nutrients you are missing, then take the next step when you are ready.

You may notice that this step is called "hyper-nourish" your body, not just nourish your body. What I mean by that is, we want to flood your body with nutrients to accelerate the healing process. For most people they are so malnourished, the body uses whatever nutrients it does get to perform the basic functions of survival. While adding in any amount of plant foods will start improving health, the results may be slow or incomplete. My method is to create an oversupply of nutrients, so the body can have access to every and any nutrient it needs for survival, and to heal and create health. You see the body instinctively wants to heal – it is programmed to heal. You see this every time you get a cut on your hand – you don't need to get out your sewing kit to close it, right? Your body closes the wound itself. It heals. Now, when people get severe chronic inflammation, like in diabetes for example, the body cannot even heal a simple wound and will develop infections that will spread dangerously and often end up needing an amputation to save their lives. No matter what disease you are suffering from, your body wants to heal, it just needs to have the right internal environment to do so: low inflammation and the right ingredients to perform the necessary tasks, nutrients!

The key to getting the maximal nourishment from plants is eating them raw. That is the best way to get the vitamins, minerals, phytoenzymes, and phytonutrients (which are good plant chemicals). A significant amount of these vital nutrients are denatured or destroyed when the food is cooked. While eating cooked vegetables and greens is totally harmless, and may provide some benefits, they do not provide the same level of rapid healing that I have witnessed using raw foods.

The most important healing food you can get is actually dark green leaves and cruciferous vegetables. Kale is an excellent green to start out with. It is extremely nutrient-dense. If kale is a bit too bitter for you to start out with, give spinach a try. Beet greens are very mild as well. Start out where you can and work your way up from there as your palate adjusts. I suggest at least four to five cups of raw greens a day.

After that, focus on getting an assortment of raw vegetables and fruits. I focus on the vegetables first since they tend to have more nutrients and less sugar. The different colors of the vegetables and fruits represent different kinds of vitamins, minerals, and other nutrients. You don't need to know what vitamins are in each plant or leaf. You should try to get in as many different colors a day as you can.

Eating your colors or "eating a rainbow" will ensure that you're doing the best for you and your health. Try to get in four to five cups of raw vegetables a day.

Now, if this is starting to feel like a huge amount of chewing, there is an easy way to get all of these raw foods in, and that is with green smoothies. To make green smoothies, you simply need a high-powered blender, I recommend Vitamix or Blendtec, and you can drink your nutrients! This has been a wonderful tool for helping people make sure they get all their nutrients in without having to think about eating them all day long. You can blend them up in the morning, put them in the refrigerator or take them to work, and know you will be nourished all day long no matter what else you choose to eat.

Another great benefit of making green smoothies is that they are easy to digest. When you make them with a high-powered blender, you don't just break the greens into smaller pieces, but you actually absorb massive amounts of nutrition at once since the cells walls are all broken apart and all of the vitamins, minerals, phytochemicals and antioxidants are released and readily absorbed into your body.

This also allows you to consume a large amount of produce at once. Far more than you can chew or swallow. When you are trying to heal from disease, try to get up to 64 ounces of smoothies throughout the day every day. You can have more as desired. There are many green smoothie recipes online, but the main component of the smoothies are greens.

Examples of these greens include:

- Beet greens
- Collard greens
- Kale
- Lacinato Kale (aka Dino Kale)
- Mustard Greens
- Rainbow Chard
- Red Chard
- Spinach
- Swiss Chard

Kale has the highest nutritional value, so I recommend that you use kale at least three days a week.

You have a great deal of greens that you can choose and start to experiment to find what you like. You can add your favorite fruits and vegetables such as cucumbers, carrots, zucchini, avocados, tomatoes, lemon, apples, oranges, pears, grapes, blueberries, bananas, and more.

You can drink them however it works best for you. I start my day off with 40 ounces for breakfast, but I did not start out that way! In the beginning it may feel like a lot of liquid, so drink as much as you can, then save the rest, and have more when you feel hungry again. Some people will drink 20 ounces three to four times a day; some need to start with six to 8 ounces at a time. The key is to drink as much as you can, as often as you need to. You may need to start with 20 ounces a day and work your way up to 64 ounces a day. This is a minimum guideline and there is no upper limit. You can have unlimited additional green smoothies all day long as often as you want.

Now notice I am talking about blending green smoothies, not juicing. While fresh juices are healthy and you can have them whenever you like, they are not whole foods; they are missing the fiber and the minerals that live in the skin of the produce. For your healing protocol, I want you to consume the whole vegetable or fruit, not just the juice.

Fresh fruits and vegetables are full of vitamins, minerals, and antioxidants. Many people are spending a ton of money buying vitamin supplements while eating foods that are making them sick. If you avoid the foods on the avoid list and start eating large volumes of fresh raw produce, you will be amazed at how much better you feel and how quickly you will feel better.

The majority of these foods should be mostly fresh and raw. Avoid frozen, cooked, steamed, and certainly avoid microwaved! Freezing, cooking, and microwaving all reduce the nutrient content of plant foods.

Most folks, when they eat vegetables, they are steamed or sautéed. They may taste great and aren't causing inflammation, but they aren't healing because the nutrients are gone. I'm not saying you shouldn't grab a pan and make a delicious plant-based meal, but it does mean that cooked foods should and do not replace your need for raw fresh plant foods. These types of foods should be the majority of your meals. When I reversed my disease, I ate eight to twelve cups a day of raw and fresh greens and vegetables a day! Back then, I hadn't discovered blending them yet, so as you can imagine, I was chomping on them all day long! I didn't really have room in my stomach for many cooked foods. I enjoyed being full and energized all day long!

Some of you may be thinking that it would be hard to have the appetite for all the other foods if you are eating that many plant foods and you are right! This is a health-improving method called crowding-out. We focus on getting all the healthy foods in and eventually we don't have the appetite or the inclination to eat the unhealthy foods. This has worked very well for clients who were resistant to giving up meat and dairy.

I am often asked about pesticides and genetically modified organisms (GMOs). Whenever possible go pesticide free because you want to avoid any toxins being introduced to your body, but it is not necessary to buy organic produce if you cannot afford it. When I first healed myself, I was a broke intern and I could not afford organic produce, yet my body still healed. I believe that the nourishment from the plant foods in the absence of inflammation and disease-causing foods provides benefits to the cells that far outweigh the potential for damage from pesticides and GMOs. I recommend going to the farmer's market if you have one near you, as they have a huge variety of fruits and vegetables that are pesticide free for a fraction of the price you pay at the supermarket. Many places have farmer's markets and other similar events so it never hurts to look around and many sellers will be happy to answer any questions that you have. I like to go 30 minutes before the farmer's market is closing and ask them for deals to buy all of their remaining produce. They will give amazing bulk discounts rather than pack up the remaining food and take it back with them.

You can eat unlimited amounts of fresh raw fruits and vegetables a day. You can eat them in any form as long as it is raw, so you have lots of room to get creative. Lemon juice or guacamole works well for salad dressing, as well as a plethora of oil-free dressings you can find by searching online.

You can even make raw vegan recipes to add some variety to your meals. There are a lot of raw vegan recipe books out there and online as well. You can also find prepared raw vegan meals in natural food stores or raw vegan restaurants.

The greatest part of your fresh vegetables should be from dark green leafy vegetables such as kale, spinach, and chard. These are great things to blend into your smoothies as well as use them in salads.

In addition to this you can have one handful of raw nuts per day. This can include raw cashews, raw almonds, or raw walnuts every day. Raw nuts are also very healthy for you. Avoid the roasted nuts as that has their nutrients lost, are salted, and are too easy to overeat. You can find raw nuts in natural food stores and many supermarkets. These nuts contain a large supply of nutrients and some, like walnuts, are also anti-inflammatory. While there has been some debate about whether raw nuts need to be soaked first, the most recent research indicates this is not necessary.[17, 20] This is because the phytates in nuts, a chemical found in seeds, has been reported past animal experiments to be an inhibitor of mineral absorption, and, therefore, it was previously recommended to soak them first to remove the phytates.[18,19] Newer human research indicates, conversely, that phytates are healthy and may be protective against osteoporosis and even cancer. [17,20,21] I sometimes soak nuts for certain recipes, since they are creamier that way, but when I eat them as a crunchy snack, I don't soak them first.

You can eat as many helpings of raw flax seeds, hemp seeds, and chia seeds as you wish. Many people like to add these to their green smoothies for a nuttier flavor, sprinkle them on salads, or make or buy raw flaxseed crackers.

If you feed your cells what they need, then they can heal, and you will feel better than ever.

Step 5:
Consume Omega-3s Every Day

By eating a healthy amount of omega-3s, I experienced some dramatic changes and within weeks my joint pain disappeared. Omega-3s contain potent anti-inflammatory properties that work at the cellular level. This is excellent for anyone who suffers from Lupus or any disease from high blood pressure to Attention-Deficit Hyperactivity Disorder (ADHD). This is because they are the ingredients to make the anti-inflammatory immune mediators PGE3 and LTB5 as you can see in the chart below. These directly and powerfully reduce inflammation in the body.

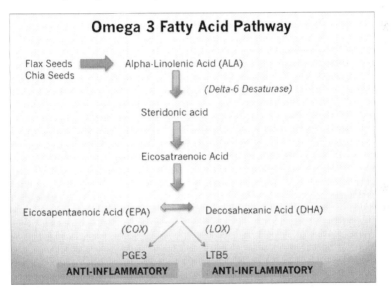

Remember, chronic inflammation is the breeding grounds for chronic disease, so these are very important to quickly reverse the inflammatory process and jump-start healing.

I have used these as a powerful tool to help people with swollen joints quickly recover range of motion and reduce pain within days.

Omega-3 fatty acids are also an important part of the membranes of your cells. They become part of the cell membrane, which improves the cellular function by making the cells more flexible and able to send and receive important messages that are necessary for basic functions and especially healing.

The issue here is that omega-3 fatty acids must be eaten in order to be present in your body. Your body cannot make them on its own. There are very few sources of omega-3 fatty acids, and most people in modern societies are severely deficient. I have found the best sources for increasing your omega-3 intake is with cold-pressed flaxseed or chia oils, as well as seaweed, flaxseeds, and chia seeds.

In the beginning, I took high doses of fish oil, but now I use plant-based products like flax seeds and chia seeds. They work extremely well, and with no risk of mercury or ocean pollutants, and have the benefits of being more ocean-friendly and sustainable.

Remember, the counterpart to omega-3 fatty acids are omega-6 fatty acids, which are responsible for creating the *inflammatory* immune mediators. Those come from oils and processed foods. When we consume omega-6 rich foods every day while neglecting the omega-3's, our bodies become massively inflamed and our health goes down the tubes.

Just by understanding these pathways, you can understand why we must both limit foods rich in omega-6 fatty acids and indulge in foods rich in omega-3 fatty acids if we want to switch our body over to a low-inflammation state and thereby initiate the healing process. I call this a "health-hack" because you can use omega-3 fatty acids to start decreasing inflammation immediately, even while inflammatory foods are still in the system, and it works.

My recommendation is to consume 1/4 cup to ½ cup of whole flax or chia seeds a day, or 2 to 3TB of cold-pressed flax or chia oil. There is no upper limit to how much you should have, base it on how you feel. Some people will get runny stools when they consume high levels of these seeds or oil because it can make your stool a bit slippery, so if your stool is very loose, you might need to titrate them slowly and spread them out over the course of your day. Realize that these are extremely healthy and necessary fats and will *not* cause you to gain weight, Rather, they increase your metabolic rate to help you reach your ideal weight.

You can soak the flax or chia seeds and eat them as a gel or grind them up in a coffee grinder as a salad topper, or use flax or chia oil in your salad dressing, but the best and easiest way to eat them is to put the whole flax seeds right into your blender when making your green smoothies. That way you have all of the nutrition you need for the entire day right in your smoothie cup. Isn't that convenient? My clients and I adore this method because it takes all the stress out of deciding what you should eat for the day. Once you consume your green smoothie with flax seeds, you are nourished! It's that easy!

Please note that you should use whole flax and chia seeds, not ground seeds nor the oils, because the omega-3 fats oxidize very quickly when exposed to air, so always grind them up right before you want to consume them.

Now, you may have heard that people do not easily convert flax and chia seeds into the anti-inflammatory Docosahexaenoic Acid (DHA) and Eicosapentaenoic Acid (EPA). This can be true, but mainly for people who consume a lot of animal products and oils. The flax and chia seeds contain an omega-3 fatty acid called alpha-linolenic acid (ALA), which requires an enzyme called Delta-6 Desaturase to convert the ALA into DHA and EPA. This very same enzyme is used in the conversion of Linoleic Acid (from vegetable oils and animal fats) into the inflammatory byproducts it creates. The enzyme appears to prefer breaking down omega-6 fatty acids. Thus, if you are consuming both omega-6 from oils and animal fats *and* flax and/or chia seeds, the enzyme will be very busy turning your omega 6 supply into inflammation and illness, instead of churning all those omega-3s into anti-inflammatory disease-busters! This is why it is essential to both eliminate the omega-6 in your diet from animal products and oils and fill up on your omega-3s. When we do this, we essentially hack into your immune system and rapidly reverse pain and inflammation.

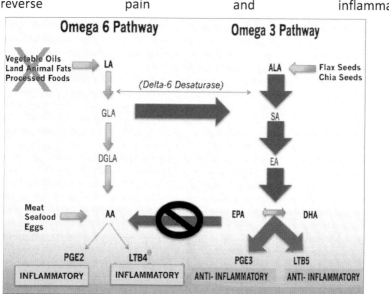

The above diagram demonstrates that when you eliminate vegetable oils, processed foods and animal fat, the Delta-6 Desaturase enzyme will be preferentially utilized by the Omega-3 pathway, which will shut down creation of further inflammatory immune cells, and instead create anti-inflammatory immune cells. The diagram also illustrates that the presence of EPA and DHA will inhibit the breakdown of Arachidonic Acid (AA) from meat and eggs into the inflammatory immune cells, which is yet another way in which Omega 3s prevent inflammation.

People often ask about fish oil as an omega 3. Indeed, fish oil is a direct source of omega 3s but my patients on it would get side effects such as easy bruising all over their bodies, and one patient even got little hemorrhages in her eyes because fish oil acts as a potent blood thinner. Fish oil is also a direct source of EPA and DHA so it bypasses your body's ability to regulate the creation of EPA and DHA the way it can with ALA. Also, there are health benefits to ALA, such as protection against dementia, that would be lost if you chose fish oil as your omega 3 supplement since it does not contain any ALA.[22]

Step 6:
Water, Water, Water!

It is of vital importance to drink lots of water. Water is essential for the majority of chemical reactions in the body to take place. This means that you can have all of the essential ingredients for your health to improve, but without enough water the necessary reactions will not take place or will happen sluggishly.

My husband and I have put countless people through our program to accelerate fitness and health, and often, when someone's results have stalled, we find they are not drinking sufficient water. We have them increase their water intake and – bam! – their results accelerate again.

Now there are conflicting arguments about how much water one really needs to consume. The Food and Drug Administration currently recommends eight glasses of water a day (8 ounces each), which is equal to 64 ounces a day, regardless of body size. In my opinion, that is barely enough to maintain health, but not nearly enough to improve health. What we have found through our clients, is that people need a minimum at least one-half of an ounce of water per pound of body weight a day, up to a gallon of water a day. That means that a person who weighs one hundred and 50 pounds should have a minimum of 75 ounces to 120 ounces (1 gallon) of water a day. A person who is two hundred pounds should have one hundred to one hundred and 20 ounces of water a day. Through repeated trials, we have discovered that that there is a rapid increase in visible results when people consume 96 ounces a day, so I usually advise people to aim for that amount as a minimum water goal if they are at 96 pounds. At this time, we are still unsure as to the mechanism of why this amount has been the optimal starting point for healing and fitness, but it is what we have repeatedly observed in our clients.

Another important function of water is to detoxify and cleanse your body. Water is absorbed in your colon, and if you do not drink enough water, your stool will be dry and hard, making it very hard to move it through your body and out. I recommend you think of your colon like an enclosed water slide. It is very difficult to go down a dry water slide, you will shimmy and twist and work very hard just to move small distances down that narrow tunnel. Now add a gushing flow of water and you fly right through the water tunnel and down the slide, no problem! I always get a big laugh when I act this out on stage! Dehydration is the most common cause of constipation, yet it is rarely addressed. I once treated a woman who had had constipation for 20 years, which had caused painful anal fissures and required two surgeries. She said I was the first doctor to ask her how much water she drank – not even the surgeons asked her! It turns out that she didn't drink any water "unless I accidentally swallow it when I brush my teeth!" After two weeks of increasing her water intake, she was able to stop the constipation medications she had been taking for 20 years. Most people, including doctors, go straight to fiber drinks and medications for constipation, but it's not necessary or helpful, it just covers up the real issue. Just by drinking your water and getting in your green smoothies, you will find that bowel movements are frequent and comfortable, the way they should be.

Dehydration is an epidemic in this country. Fascinatingly, the most common symptom of dehydration is a lack of thirst. So, if you are severely dehydrated, then you aren't thirsty. It sounds like a paradox, but it is most likely a coping mechanism for the body, so you don't suffer from thirst in a drought. Once people start drinking a lot of water, as I encourage you to do, they notice they feel thirsty quite frequently. The drive to drink comes back online and you experience the normal desire to drink water.

Since you already will be in the bathroom quite a lot with all of that fiber from the raw foods, the water will only increase that time with the improved bowel movements, and also the bladder trying to cope with all of the increased flow! Your body will adjust, and if this is a huge change for you, I suggest you increase it more slowly, start with aiming for 1/2 ounce per pound of your body weight and working your way up.

I also recommend you get all of your water in by early evening, so you aren't waking up all night to urinate!

When I healed, I drank a gallon of water a day. Before that, I was having maybe one or two glasses of water a day, relying on diet soda, coffee, and energy drinks to keep up my energy as an intern at the hospital. Remarkably, when I nourished my body and drank my water, I no longer needed caffeine; my body had the fuel to keep me alert and active all day long.

I recommend you stay away from alcohol and coffee while you are healing; they slow down the healing process and interfere with opportunities to drink water. If you are addicted to caffeine, you can wean yourself off slowly or at least switch to green tea which has some anti-inflammatory properties. Realize that caffeine is a diuretic, which means it causes you to urinate more and lose precious water, so if you drink caffeine, you need to compensate with more water.

Integrating the Steps

I ate this way, and my blood work has been negative for 10 years. I have been off medications for nine years and I am completely healthy.

According to most medicine this shouldn't have happened – yet it did! Modern medicine hasn't quite caught up to the healing properties of this type of eating.

Our cells are highly flexible and can recover from many great insults if we avoid things that hurt them and give them what they need to heal.

Our diet is the major culprit to what causes inflammation in our bodies and disease. Believe it or not, genetics only account for roughly three to 5 percent of inflammation and disease.

Because of this we really are what we eat. We can eat vibrant living foods and be vibrantly healthy, or eat processed, toxic foods and be sluggish, obese, and chronically ill.

We are currently facing a health crisis of epidemic proportions. We are witnessing the first generation of children that are not expected to outlive their parents.

This is because we are getting fatter than ever and sicker than ever at younger and younger ages. Type II diabetes was called, "Adult-Onset Diabetes" when I was in medical school, but now it is called Type II Diabetes because it is so common in children.

We are seeing more and more illnesses develop in children, including obesity, high blood pressure, heart disease, Cancer, ADHD, bipolar illness, Autism, and Depression and countless others. I strongly believe that these are not caused by separate processes but are instead symptoms of a larger problem: food children are eating today! Most children are eating exorbitant amounts of fast food, dairy products, meats, and processed foods *at every meal*, rarely if ever eating fresh whole healthy foods. Then they wash them down with sodas, sugary drinks, or energy drinks, ignoring their growing bodies' need for precious water. This is why they are the sickest generation in history and it's only getting worse. There is no greater travesty in my eyes than watching our children get sick and die before our eyes; we must do something, we must.

Convenience has been used as an excuse to damage and poison our own food supply. Now we are being forced to pay the piper.

It does not have to be that way anymore. You can change your eating habits and improve your life and health. You can save your children from every becoming sick. It's never too late to start making important changes!

Inspiration to change

There is a Chinese proverb that says, "He who takes medication and neglects his food wastes the skill of his doctor."

It is important for you to do your part, too.

If you really wish to kick-start your health start looking into foods that are called "superfoods." Superfoods are foods with abnormally high levels of nutrients in them. Some examples are cacao, goji berries, maca powder, chlorella, and spirulina. These are great additions to a healthy diet. My favorite is cacao, which is raw chocolate before it is destroyed by adding cow's milk and processing it. I love to take cacao, almond milk, a banana and run it through a blender. It's what we call "chocolate milk" in my house. It's a super healthy drink that is much better for you than something that is processed.

You can enjoy delicious foods while eating a whole foods plant-based diet.

If I want ice cream I take frozen bananas, almond milk, a splash of vanilla and blend them until it turns into soft serve. It's a healthier alternative that does not attack your health.

If you aren't sure on where to start recipe-wise, there are many easy to find recipes online that you can print out and try. If you look up whole foods plant-based diet online you can find lots of recipes, videos, and even cookbooks.

Frequently Asked Questions

Taking back your health is not just a dietary change – it's a lifestyle change. With any change, I'm sure you have a lot of questions. Here are the top 7 questions I get asked on a regular basis. Don't worry. Feel free to ask them again. I'm always ready, willing, and able to help.

1 - Is eating plant-based foods boring?

Foods taste better without being covered in all the junk we think makes them taste better. Plant-based, raw foods are absolutely delicious when you give them a chance to shine on their own instead of trying to hide their natural goodness under layers of butter, margarine, sour cream, etc. You'll notice food tastes different when it's free of all the extra fat and processed flavors. And I don't mean different bad; I mean different good. That being said, it takes time to reeducate your palate. From my experience, it takes about two weeks for people to stop craving the foods they were addicted to and start appreciating the nuanced and delicious flavors in plant foods. There are also many exciting ways to prepare them. In my video, *Super Healthy Meals for Your Family*, I teach a gang of skeptical moms how to make super easy, healthy, and fast, raw dishes for breakfast, lunch, dinner, and dessert, that the whole family will love. The feedback I have gotten is that they never knew how good raw food could be!

2 - Will I have low energy if I only eat plant-based foods?

Low energy is an epidemic in our country. The producers of coffee and high-caffeine drinks are profiting wildly from it. The issue is that people do not have a caffeine deficiency. They have a nutrient deficiency. People who switch to a plant-based diet notice their energy levels are more consistent than any other time in their life. Plus, it's not an energy that waxes, wanes or crashes. It's consistent. Think of high-fiber and nutrient-heavy foods as the fire that burn for hours versus the low-fiber and nutrient-light foods extinguish in a flash. People who use the hyper-nourishing plan that I teach, rich in raw foods, tell me that they have more energy than they can ever remember. Many have given up coffee because they find they just don't need it anymore.

3 - Can I get enough calcium eating a plant-based diet?

A diverse, plant-based diet is one of the best sources of calcium you'll find without the unhealthy effects of dairy. Americans have such a high rate of osteoporosis isn't because we're not getting enough dietary calcium, but we're consuming an excess of animal protein, which leaches calcium from the bones. The best, most well-absorbed source of calcium for humans comes from leafy greens like broccoli and kale.

4 - Can carbs make me fat?

Carbohydrates have gotten a bad reputation, and undeservedly so. When most people think of carbs, they are envisioning processed carbohydrates like processed breads, pastas, and cakes. Realize though, all vegetables, beans, and fruits are sources of carbohydrates – good healthy carbohydrates! What I am teaching you in this book, is the key to superior health comes from eating a very high carbohydrate diet. It's important to understand that carbohydrates are your body's primary fuel source. They manage your heart rate, digestion, breathing, exercising, walking, and thinking. From the research that Thomas Tadlock and I have performed on thousands of clients, we have discovered that the more raw greens and vegetables a person consumes, the faster their metabolism is, and the more fat they burn. When I am preparing for a fitness photoshoot, I double the amount of green smoothies I drink, in addition to my other foods, to ramp up the nourishment and get my metabolism to even higher levels. When it comes to healthy carbohydrates, the more you eat, the less fat you have.

5 - Are plant proteins complete proteins?

The old idea of needing to eat "complete proteins" has been disproven for many years. In fact, Plant proteins are as complete as you can find. The American Dietetic Association's position statement reads: "Plant sources of protein alone can provide adequate amounts of the essential and nonessential amino acids, assuming that dietary protein sources from plants are reasonably varied and that caloric intake is sufficient to meet energy needs. Whole grains, legumes, vegetables, seeds, and nuts all contain essential and nonessential amino acids."

6 - Can I get enough protein eating a plant-based diet?

You'd be surprised at the amount of protein you find in whole, natural plant-based foods. Spinach is 51 percent protein; mushrooms, 35 percent; beans, 26 percent; oatmeal, 16 percent; whole wheat pasta, 15 percent; corn, 12 percent; and potatoes, 11 percent. The average American consumes over 100 grams of protein a day. This is a dangerous amount. The meat industry has propagated a myth that the human body needs animal proteins when they are actually some of the worst things for our health. Our body can get plenty of proteins from an abundance of plant foods. If you eat whole plant foods to fullness, you will get enough protein for health. Protein supplements are not necessary and are discouraged because they are often processed or contain milk derivatives and sugars. By eating a plant-strong diet, you get just the right amount of protein.

7. What about caffeine?

Caffeine is being used more and more by our culture. If we have no energy, we often take something with caffeine in it to get ourselves through our days. This is actually a symptom of malnourishment since *food* should be supplying our energy, not caffeine. Along with being a stimulant that can easily be abused, caffeine can be very inflammatory and, therefore, should be avoided.

An exception is green tea, which has some anti-inflammatory properties. A cup of green tea a day is probably okay for you if you feel the need to have something. Do your best to avoid coffee, energy drinks, and other things that have a great amount of caffeine in them.

During this time, you may go through caffeine withdrawal, which includes fatigue, headaches, and cloudy thinking. The withdrawal symptoms will fade after about two weeks. When I stopped all caffeine, I had headaches for about two weeks. Not fun, but after they wore off, I began to feel more energetic overall. If you do the same, then you should feel the same in about the same amount of time. If you use a lot of caffeinated products, consider weaning yourself off a bit more slowly or switch over to green tea, to mitigate the withdrawal symptoms.

Interestingly, I have had many people say they went off their coffee on their own after starting to drink 40 ounces of green smoothie in the morning because their energy was so high, they no longer craved it.

8. What about alcohol?

Your best bet is to avoid it. When you are feeling better and maintaining your health, it is most likely okay to have a glass of wine here or there when you're feeling better. However, for now, it's best to avoid it so your body can focus itself on recovery.

9. What about gluten?

If you have a diagnosed sensitivity to gluten, it's best to avoid it. Gluten is found in wheat, rye, and barley. You will find it in foods like traditional breads and pasta. I believe that most people who believe they have gluten sensitivity really are reacting to processed grains. If you want to eat whole unprocessed grains but are worried about sensitivity, try going completely off gluten-containing products for a few weeks and then gradually try reintroducing them when you are feeling better and see how you feel. I personally do not have a gluten sensitivity, but there is a high percentage of people with Lupus who do. It is not necessary, however, to consume grains for this healing protocol. I have not found it to have healing properties and consider it a health-maintenance foods rather than a healing food.

10. Do I need any supplements?

This is a whole food approach to healing, so no other vitamins are required to start nourishing your cells and begin the healing process. That being, said, at this point, the newest research indicates that many people suffer from a dysfunctional gut from the effects of meat, dairy and processed foods on their healthy bacteria and gut wall. For this reason, it is often helpful to add a high-grade probiotic during the first couple months of changing your diet, which will help digestion and maximize the benefits you receive from eating well.

I do not personally take a B12 supplement, which is currently a hot topic in the vegan world, but I do enjoy the flavors in nutritional yeast, which is usually fortified with B vitamins, and my B12 levels are usually very high, most likely from enjoying my nutritional yeast so much. The normal levels of B12 are debated because they were measured in people who eat the standard diet that has a lot of meat, so they are really just typical levels in healthy-appearing meat-eaters, but are not necessarily the levels our body actually needs. Most people I know that eat vegan or plant-based diets take supplemental B12, "just in case", but I know many vibrantly healthy people who do not take any B12. At this point, I think it's a personal decision – and one that is easy to change if you feel it is necessary.

Favorite Recipes

These are some recipes from my kitchen. Feel free to change them up according to your taste. You may like it sweeter and want to add more fruit or dates, or you may want to add some fresh herbs. You can also change up the greens depending on your tastes and what you have available, like kale, spinach, mustard greens chard, dandelion green romaine lettuce, etc. Kale is the most nutrient-dense and should be a frequent player in the rotation. If you don't have (or like) all of the ingredients, make a substitution or simply leave it out.

I encourage you to try your own recipes out too, just make sure the main ingredient is fresh greens and then add your own fruits and vegetables to taste. If you mess up and the taste isn't quite what you like, I have found adding bananas and/or almond milk is a miracle fix for bitter smoothies. Also, the stems of kale and other greens tend to be bitter, so I recommend you remove them and just use the leaves.

You might want to start out with sweeter smoothies as you adjust to the taste of the greens. You will likely find that with time you start enjoying the taste of the greens and cut back on your fruits, which is more ideal. I usually add chlorella and spirulina to my smoothies, super nutritious superfoods, but they are not necessary if you don't have access to them.

Remember to use fresh, raw ingredients, organic whenever possible. Frozen foods lose a lot of their nutrients and are not as healthy and revitalizing. Some people like to add frozen foods as a flavoring, like a frozen banana, and this is OK as long as you realize that does not count toward your total plant intake for the day. Make sure your produce is fresh and ripe and make sure you remove any brown spots before blending.

Unless specified otherwise, add filtered water to the listed ingredients until you reach 3/4 way to the top of the vegetables in the blender, add five to six ice cubes and blend for about two minutes or until fully liquefied.

If you use fresh wheatgrass, add at least a cup of ice and blend for five minutes to blend up the fibrous grass. These blend times are meant for the Vitamix blender. If you are using a lower grade blender, you will have to blend longer, and determine the times on your own with practice.

If you like a thinner consistency, use more water. For creamy smoothies add avocado and/or bananas. You can also use nut milks or coconut water if you prefer. Some store-bought nut milks are sweetened with cane sugar, so try to find sugar free (or make your own). Do not add sugar to your smoothie or other foods; instead use fruits and dates or other sweet fruits to achieve sweetness.

Green smoothies can be stored in the refrigerator for up to 24 hours. When they are left out, they degrade quickly. I usually add ice to my travel jars in addition to packing them in a cold storage box with ice packs to ensure freshness on the go.

Due to high demand for healing and tasty green smoothie recipes, I created a recipe book called *Green Smoothie Recipes to Kick-Start Health & Healing*. I included six of my favorite recipes from that book for you here so you can get started experiencing just how delicious healing can be!

The Beginner

This tasty smoothie makes a great first smoothie.

6 cups kale leaves

1 pear

1 large banana

1 cup of pineapple

1 avocado

Add almond milk ½ the way to the top of veggies

Add filtered water to the listed ingredients until you reach ¾ way to the top of the food in the blender, add 5 to 6 ice cubes and blend for about two minutes or until fully liquefied.

Note: These blend times are meant for the Vitamix blender. If you are using a lower grade blender, you will have to blend longer and determine the times on your own with practice.

Rise and Shine Smoothie

Way better for you than orange juice and delicious all day long.

5 tangerines (or 2 large oranges) peel removed

1 banana

2 carrots

6 cups green kale

Optional: 3000mg Chlorella

Add filtered water to the listed ingredients until you reach ¾ way to the top of the vegetables in the blender, add 5 to 6 ice cubes and blend for about two minutes or until fully liquefied.

Note: These blend times are meant for the Vitamix blender. If you are using a lower grade blender, you will have to blend longer and determine the times on your own with practice.

Chocolate Green Dream

To satisfy your sweet tooth. This is known by my son as "chocolate milk" in my house.

¼ cup cacao powder

1 cup almond milk

1 cup filtered water

2 dates

1 avocado

6 cups collard green leaves

1 banana

Add filtered water to the listed ingredients until you reach ¾ way to the top of the vegetables in the blender, add 5 to 6 ice cubes and blend for about two minutes or until fully liquefied.

Note: These blend times are meant for the Vitamix blender. If you are using a lower grade blender, you will have to blend longer and determine the times on your own with practice.

Green and Grape

The perfect amount of sweetness makes this smoothie a household favorite!

2 cups red grapes

2 large bananas

6 cups spinach

4 ice cubes

Add filtered water to the listed ingredients until you reach ¾ way to the top of the vegetables in the blender, add 5 to 6 ice cubes and blend for about two minutes or until fully liquefied.

Note: These blend times are meant for the Vitamix blender. If you are using a lower grade blender, you will have to blend longer and determine the times on your own with practice.

Orange You Refreshed?

A delicious drink for citrus fans!

6 tangerines, peeled

2 carrots (unpeeled)

Juice of 1 large lemon

1 avocado

6 cups black kale

4 ice cubes

Add filtered water to the listed ingredients until you reach ¾ way to the top of the vegetables in the blender, add 5 to 6 ice cubes and blend for about two minutes or until fully liquefied.

Note: These blend times are meant for the Vitamix blender. If you are using a lower grade blender, you will have to blend longer and determine the times on your own with practice.

Omega Sunrise

6 cups kale

3 oranges

1 banana

¼ cup Chia seeds

4 ice cubes

Add filtered water to the listed ingredients until you reach ¾ way to the top of the vegetables in the blender, add 5 to 6 ice cubes and blend for about two minutes or until fully liquefied.

Note: These blend times are meant for the Vitamix blender. If you are using a lower grade blender, you will have to blend longer and determine the times on your own with practice.

Here are some fun healing recipes I like to make. I encourage you to look up raw vegan recipes online or check out some raw food books.

Thomas' Raw Banana Cream Cereal

This is a creamy and sweet protein-packed breakfast treat that will more than satisfy your craving for cold cereal and milk. You can experiment with ingredients, such as switching out raisins for chopped dates or skipping the coconut. The combination of bananas, nuts, and almond milk really hits the spot. It's also one of only three delicious things my husband has ever made.

Ingredients:

1 cup raw almonds (or any raw nut)

¼ cup canned or boxed coconut milk (mix well to get creamy even texture)

1 whole banana sliced

¼ cup raisins

¼ cup dried or fresh coconut (optional)

1 cup almond milk

Chop peanuts in food processor until finely chopped. Pour into a large bowl. Add sliced bananas, coconut, and raisins. Add coconut cream. Add Almond milk until the desired level as you would with cold cereal.

Superfood Green Energy Bars

I always keep these in the refrigerator. They are great for breakfast or anytime and easy to keep with you.

Ingredients:

¾ cup raw almonds, soaked at least 1 hour and drained

1 cup dates, pitted and soaked at least 1 hour

¼ cup raw sunflower seeds soaked at least 1 hour and drained

¼ cup goji berries

¼ cup raw cacao nibs

¼ cup almond butter or tahini

½ cup raisins soaked in 1 cup water for at least 1 hour (save soak water).

2 Tbsp. flax seeds soaked in 1/4 cup water for at least 1 hour

1 ½ Tsp. cacao powder

1 ½ Tsp. chlorella powder

¼ Tsp. cinnamon

1 pinch cardamom

½ cup Shredded coconut

1. Drain almonds and dates and process into chunks in a food processor fitted with an S-blade. Add to a large bowl. Add sunflower seeds, goji berries, cacao nibs, almond butter (or tahini), raisins, raisin soak water, flax seeds, carob powder, spirulina powder, cinnamon, and cardamom. If you are using a dehydrator, add coconut. If you are refrigerating, save coconut until the end. Mix thoroughly for a couple of minutes.

2. If dehydrating, flatten onto a Teflex-lined dehydrator tray until it's ¼ inch thick. Dehydrate at 110 degrees for 6 hours. Flip over and remove the Teflex paper. Dehydrate for another 6-8 hours. Should be chewy.

3. If not dehydrating form into 2-inch balls and roll in shredded coconut (if using). Chill in refrigerator for at least 30 minutes.

Dr. G's Raw Donut Holes

These taste somewhere between donuts and macaroons. Really yummy.

1 cup shredded coconut

1/3 cup raw walnuts

1/2 Tsp. vanilla

1/4 Tsp. cinnamon

1 pinch sea salt

4 dates (pits removed)

1 Tbsp. cacao powder (optional)

2 Tsp maple syrup

Use a food processor to process shredded coconut for about 20 seconds.

Add walnuts, vanilla, cinnamon, and salt. Process until another 30 secs or until nuts well broken down.

Add dates, cacao and maple syrup and process until it begins to clump.

Form the dough into 1" balls.

Dehydrate at 105 degrees for 1 hour to warm and set. If you don't have a dehydrator, set out in the sun for 3 hours. Refrigerate leftovers.

Almond Butter and Apple Sandwich

Great for a fun alternative to a sandwich. Children love them too!

Ingredients:

1 organic apple

raw almond butter

organic raisins

Slice an apple into thin rounds.

Apply Almond Butter to each apple slice

Add a layer of raisins to one slice

Top with a second slice and squeeze them together so they stick.

Repeat. Most apples make 3-4 sandwiches.

Raw Macaroons

Mash a banana with a fork

Roll into 1" balls

Roll each banana ball in shredded coconut, then in cacao powder.

Refrigerate for at least an hour or overnight to firm up.

Dr. G's Raw Chocolate Chia Seed Pudding

2 Tbsp. chia seeds
½ cup almond milk (or nondairy milk of your choice)
2 Tbsp. maple syrup
1 Tbsp. cacao powder
½ Tsp. vanilla extract

Combine all the ingredients

Stir or whisk all the ingredients together and leave on countertop for 20 minutes.
Stir again after 20 minutes.
You want all of the chocolate to dissolve.
Refrigerate 4-6 hours or overnight to thicken.

Dr. G's Living Lasagna

This is a favorite at dinner time. Much better if you can make 1 day in advance and refrigerate overnight.

Ingredients:

¼ cup basil

3 ½ cups macadamia nuts

1 ¾ Tsp. salt

1 Tsp. fresh ground black pepper

3 Tsp. and 1/4 cup apple cider vinegar

1 ½ cups filtered water

4 Roma tomatoes

1 Tsp. minced oregano

6 Tbsp. + 2 TB filtered water

1 Tbsp. rosemary

1 large zucchini thinly sliced lengthwise

1 large yellow squash thinly sliced lengthwise

1 bunch kale

4 large tomatoes, sliced

To make "Cheese": Take ½ cup basil, 3 cups macadamia nuts, ½ Tsp. salt, ¼ Tsp. black pepper, 3 Tsp. apple cider vinegar. Process in food processor with s blade with up to 1 ½ cup filtered water if needed until ricotta consistency.

To make Sauce: Blend enough Roma tomatoes until you reach 2 cup mark on the blender. Add ½ cup macadamia nuts, ¼ cup basil, 1 Tsp. oregano, ¼ cup apple cider vinegar, 1 Tsp. salt, ½ Tsp. black pepper, 6 Tbsp. filtered water, 1Tbsp. rosemary, blend on high 30 sec until smooth.

Toss zucchini and squash with 2 TB water and ¼ Tsp. salt. Marinate for an hour. If you have a dehydrator, dehydrate at 110 for an hour for softer noodles.

Lightly oil bottom of a square baking pan using spray bottle of olive oil. Put down a layer of kale, then a layer of zucchini, then layer of sliced tomato, then half of the ricotta and half the sauce. Repeat the layers.

Can be served immediately, suggest refrigerating overnight. If you have a dehydrator, it tastes fabulous if you dehydrate it at 110 for a couple of hours to warm it up (without cooking it) and congeal the flavors. If you don't have a dehydrator and would like it warmer, you can take it out of the refrigerator and let it warm up to room temperature before serving or eat it cold.

<u>Dr. G's Crunchy Kale Chips</u>

Satisfy your chip cravings without sacrificing your health!

Ingredients:

2 bunches of kale, rinse and remove stem

¼ cup lemon juice

Sea salt to taste

¼ cup of nutritional yeast (more or less to taste)

Instructions:

Mix the lemon juice, salt, and yeast in a large mixing bowl.

Tear, or roughly chop the kale leaves up into chip size pieces. Toss the kale pieces into the bowl with the yeast mixture. Massage into the kale.

Spread kale out on dehydrator trays.

Dehydrate 5-6 hours at 115 degrees until completely dry and crunchy.

Serve immediately. Store remaining kale chips in a glass jar, eat within 2 days.

Photo Album

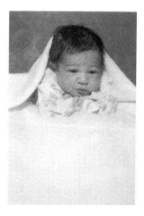

Two weeks old, 1977 Bayside, New York

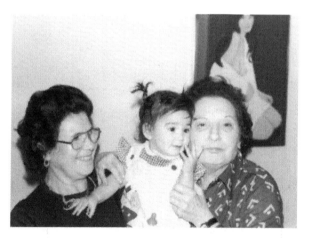

9 months old, with my Grandmother Adele Orlowski (left) and Great-Grandmother Rose Rosenberg (right).

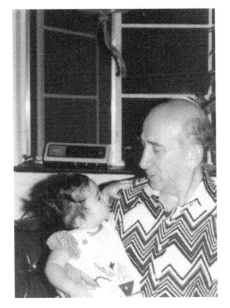

9 months old, with my favorite Grandfather, Solomon Orlowski

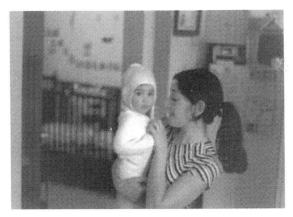

14 months-old with my mother, Gina Goldner, Bayside, New York 1977

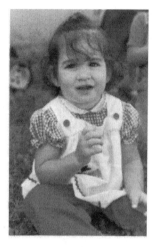

2 Years old, Bayshore, NY, 1979

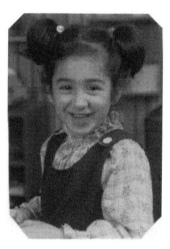

Four years-old, Hicksville, New York 1981

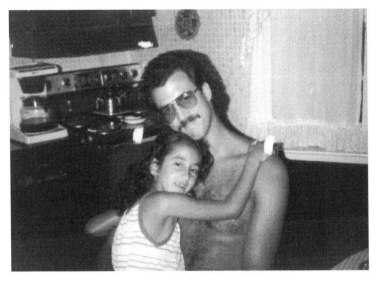

7 years old with father, Allan Goldner, Hicksville, NY 1984.

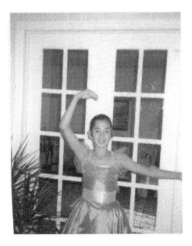

10 years old Dance Recital, Westchester, PA, 1987

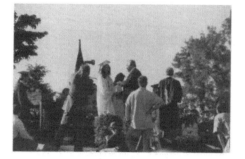

High School Graduation 1995.

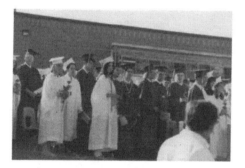

After two years of chemotherapy and multiple other medications, I managed to graduate in the top 10 of my high school class and graduated with honors... and a round moon face from all of the steroids!

Medical School Temple University School of Medicine at West Penn Hospital, 2002

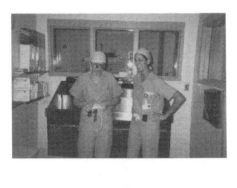

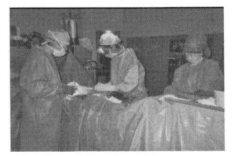

I had lost a lot of weight from stress, and soon after these photographs were taken, I developed anti-cardiolipin antibodies, which led to blood clots and a mini-stroke, but I was always grateful to be there following my dream to become a doctor.

Medical School Graduation

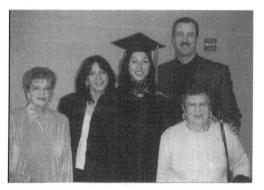

Temple University School of Medicine Class of 2004

All smiles with my parents and 2 grandmothers at my medical school graduation.

Back on medication and at my heaviest weight, but full of happiness, gratitude, and love.

The Day before our wedding, Twin Falls, Maui 2005

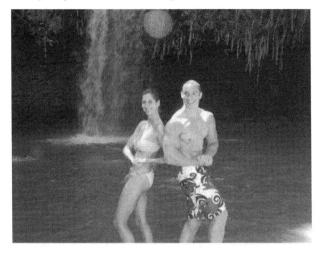

Getting Maui'd! October 5, 2005

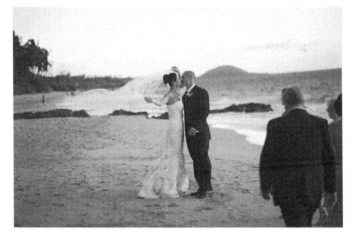

The man who changed everything, Thomas Tadlock

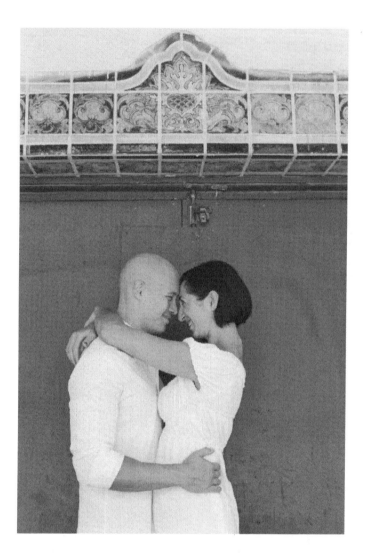

With my husband, Thomas Tadlock, 2011

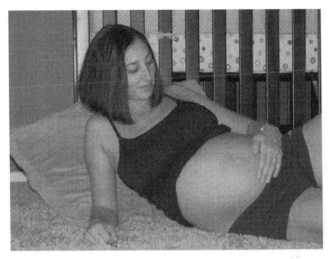

The Next Miracle Man in My life

9 months pregnant with my first son, Solomon, 2009. Everyone was terrified that pregnancy would bring back my disease, but I felt at happy and at peace.

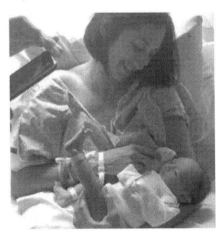

02/02/2009 Solomon was born! He was healthy and so was I. I cried every time I looked at his beautiful face.

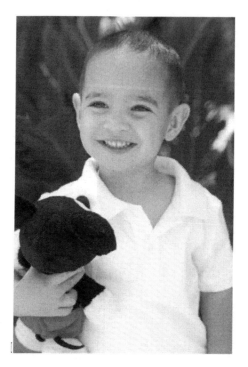

My first-born son, Solomon, at 2 years old, 2011

My Role Models and Biggest Supporters

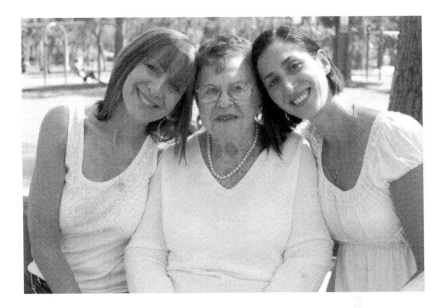

My Mother Regina Goldner (left), my grandmother Adele Orlowski (middle) and me (right), 2011.

Miracle #2 on the way – My second son, Alexander!

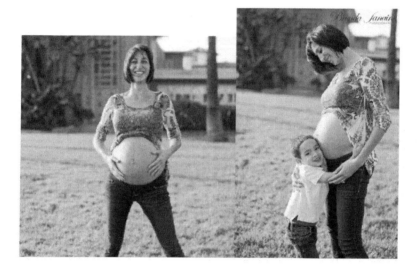

4 days away from baby #2, with Solomon, 2012

Nobody blinked an eye when I got pregnant this time, even my doctors were confident that I was healthy by now!

My Second Son, Alexander

Alexander has brought so much laughter and joy.

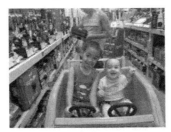

He is much like his mother, he always seems happy just to be alive!

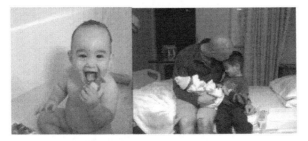

Alex born 12/17/2012

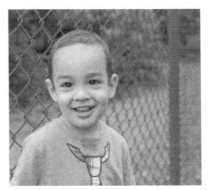

2 years old, 2014

2012 Vegan Health & Fitness Magazine Feature on Healthy Vegan Families

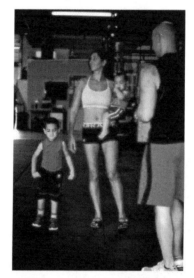

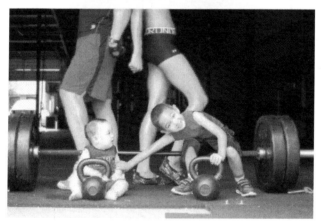

Feature in Vegan Health & Fitness Magazine 2012

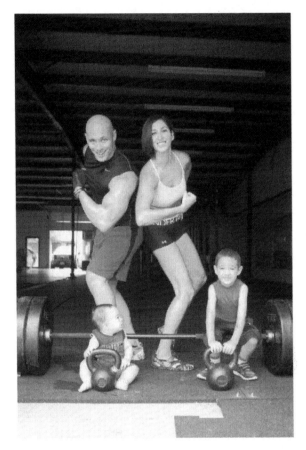

My second son Alex was only 5 months old when we did this photoshoot – my first ever photoshoot in exercise clothing. It was a big honor but definitely nerve-wracking!

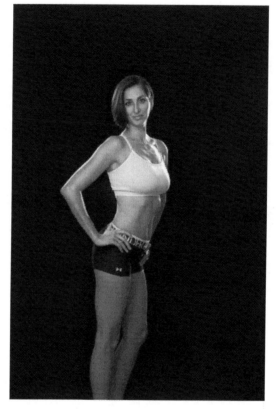

vGirls 2012

Photo by Melissa Schwartz who created a popular campaign called vGirls/vGuys to showcase how healthy and strong people can be on a 100% Vegan Diet.

I was pretty nervous about a close-up in so little clothing, but Melissa was fantastic and helped me pose. This photograph was taken when my second son Alex was 9 months old.

My Family, Cover of Vegan Health & Fitness Magazine
November/December 2014 Issue

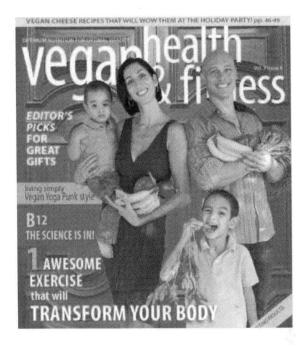

In 2014, Vegan Health & Fitness Magazine featured our family on the front cover! Inside were two articles about my family and how my Husband and I manage a wonderful family life and our mission to teach people how to heal and grow old with the person they love.

There is also an article by me called, "Plant-Based Cheese, The Vegan Holy Grail," which has my best recipes for healthier vegan cheeses!

Featured in the upcoming Documentary "Whitewashed 2015

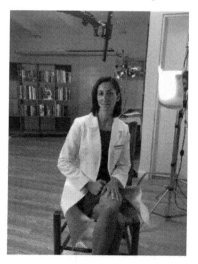

The face I make when an interviewer asks me if you need milk for calcium!

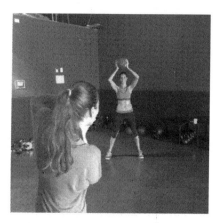

Getting documentary footage of me working out, healthy and strong!

Featured in the upcoming Documentary "Eating You Alive" about dramatic health transformations from eating a plant-based diet.

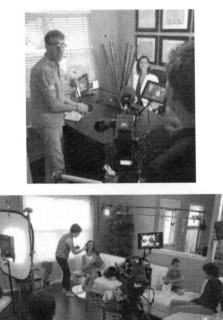

The film crew was so sweet and truly on an inspired mission to heal the world.

They also cleaned up so well before they left, it was like they were never there!

The 3rd Annual International Plant-Based Nutrition Healthcare Conference 2015

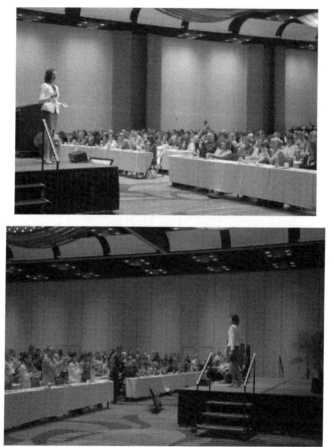

Teaching 600+ healthcare professionals how to heal autoimmune disease with supermarket foods at the 3rd Annual Plant-Based Nutrition Healthcare Conference, 2015. I was honored to receive a standing ovation.

Thank you for purchasing this book. I hope it brings you great health and hope.

For a special bonus please go here:

http://GoodbyeLupus.com/BookBonus

For more information about treatment, upcoming events, or to get a zoom, facetime, or phone consultation, go to my website:

http://www.GoodbyeLupus.com

Make sure you follow me on social media for free information, inspiration and Q&A sessions.

Instagram: @GoodbyeLupus

Facebook: @GoodbyeLupus

YouTube: youtube.com/brookegoldnermd

I wish you amazing fitness and health!

Dr. G

Citations

1. Chang, Eugene. June 5, 2012. Dietary-fat-induced taurocholic acid promotes pathobiont expansion and colitis in Il10$^{-/-}$ mice. *Nature.* June 2012; 487: 104–108.

2. Campbell, T., & Campbell, T. (2005). *The China study: The most comprehensive study of nutrition ever conducted and the startling implications for diet, weight loss and long-term health.* Dallas, Tex.: BenBella Books.

3. Larsson, Susanna C., Orsini, Nicola. Red Meat and Processed Meat Consumption and All-Cause Mortality: A Meta- Analysis. *Am. J. Epidemiol.* Oct. 2013; 179 (3), 282-289

4. Campbell, PT. May 2009. Mismatch repair polymorphisms and risk of colon cancer, tumor microsatellite instability and interactions with lifestyle factors. *Gut.* May 2009; 58(5), 661-667

5. Rohrmann, Sabine. Meat and dairy consumption and the Subsequent Cancer in a U.S. Cohort Study. *Cancer Causes Control* 2007; 18: 41-50

6. Moschos SJ, Mantzoros CS. The role of the IGF system in cancer: from basic to clinical studies and clinical applications. *Oncology.* 2002;63(4):317-32.

7. Rincon M, Rudin E, Barzilai N. The insulin/IGF-1 signaling in mammals and its relevance to human longevity. *Exp Gerontol.* 2005 Nov. ;40(11):873-7.

8. Sharpe R. Are oestrogens involved in falling sperm counts and disorders of the male reproductive tract? *Lancet* 341:1392, 1993.

9. Janowski T. Mammary secretion of oestrogens in the cow. *Domest Anim Endocrinol.* July 2002; 23 (1-2):125-37.

10. Abelow B. Cross-cultural association between dietary animal

protein and hip fracture: a hypothesis. *Calcific Tissue Int* 50:14-8, 1992.

11. Frassetto LA. Worldwide incidence of hip fracture in elderly women: relation to consumption of animal and vegetable foods. *J Gerontol A Biol Sci Med Sci.* Oct. 2000; 55(10):M585-92.

12. Saukkonen T, Virtanen SM, Karppinen M, et al. Significance of cow's milk protein antibodies as risk factor for childhood IDDM: interaction with dietary cow's milk intake and HLA-DQB1 genotype. Childhood Diabetes in Finland Study Group. *Dibetologia.* 1998;41:72–78.

13. Kimpimaki T, Erkkola M, Korhonen S, et al. Short-term exclusive breastfeeding predisposes young children with increased genetic risk of type I diabetes to progressive beta-cell autoimmunity. *Diabetologia.* 2001;44:63–69.

14. Rueda-Clausen, CF et al. Olive, Soybean, and Palm Oils Intake Have a Similar Acute Detrimental Effect Over the Endothelial Function in Healthy Young Subjects. *Nutr Metab Cardiovasc Dis.* 2007; 17 (1): 50-7

15. Jenkins, David JA et al. Glycemic Index: Overview of Implications in Health and Disease. *Am J Clinical Nutrition* July 2002; 76 (1) 266S-273S

16. Masters, Rachel, et al. Whole and Refined Grain Intakes Are Related to Inflammatory Protein Concentrations in Human Plasma. *The Journal of Nutrition.* March 2010; 140 (3): 587-594

17. Urbano, G. et al. The Role of Phytic Acid in Legumes: Antinutrient or Beneficial Function? *J. Physiolo. Biochem. 2000; 56 (3): 283-295*

18. Mellanby, Edward. The Rickets-Producing And Anti-Calcifying Action of Phytate. *J. Physiol.* 1949; 109: 488-533

19. House, William A, Welch, Ross M, Van Campen, Darrel R. Effect of Phytic Acid n the Absorption, Distribution, and Endogenous Excretion of Zinc in Rats. *J. Nutr.* 1982; 112: 941-953

20. Walker, A. R. P., Fox, F. W., Irving, J. T. Studies in Human Mineral Metabolism: The Effect of Bread Rich in Phytate Phosphorus on the Metabolism of Certain Mineral Salts with Special Reference to Calcium. *Biochem J.* 1948; 42(3): 452–462.

21. Lopez-Gonzalez, A.A. et al. Phytate (*myo*)-Inositol Hexaphosphate) and Risk Factors for Osteoporosis. *J Med Food* 2008; 11 (4): 747-752

22. Kazumasa Yamagishi et al, Serum α-linolenic and other ω-3 fatty acids, and risk of disabling dementia: Community-based nested case–control study. Clin Nutr. 2016 May 24. pii: S0261-5614(16)30106-6.

Made in the USA
Columbia, SC
09 March 2023

13544084R00061